WHAT'S YOUR POTION?

Liquid Refreshments to Nourish Body, Mind & Spirit

By Morwyn

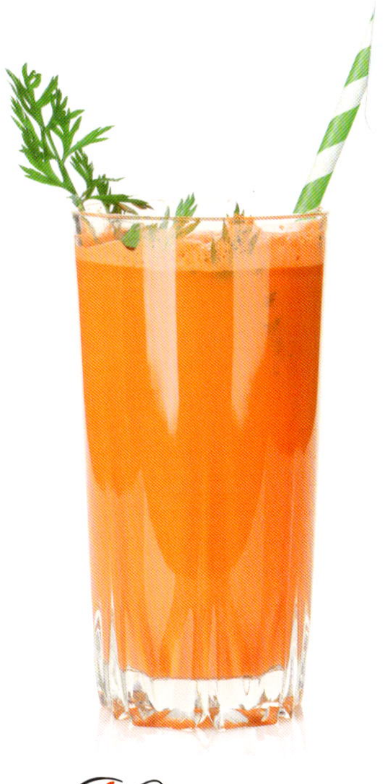

Schiffer Publishing Ltd

4880 Lower Valley Road • Atglen, PA 19310

Other Schiffer Books by Morwyn

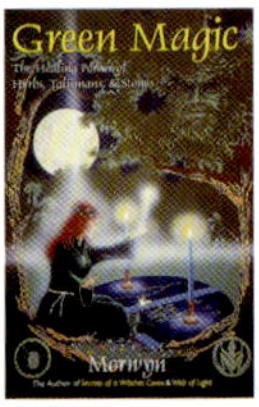

Green Magic:
The Healing Power
of Herbs, Talismans,
& Stones
978-0-924608-18-6

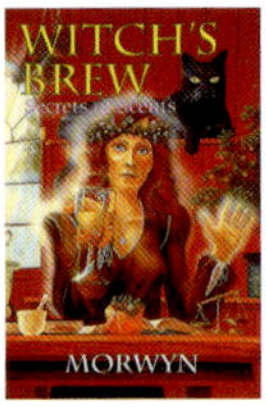

Witch's Brew:
Secrets of Scents
978-0-924608-19-3

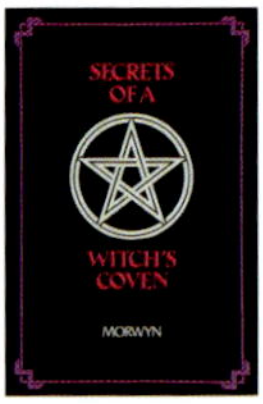

Secrets of a
Witch's Coven
978-0-914918-80-6

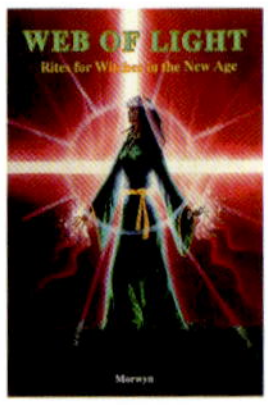

Web of Light:
Rites for Witches
in the New Age
978-0-924608-17-9

Note: The information presented herein is not meant to substitute for professional medical care. If you are suffering from a malady, see your health care professional. © for unmarked images goes to the following: A K Choudhury. Andrii Gorulko. angelsimon. bloodua. chviroj. Denira777. Digidesign. digitalr. eAlisa. egal. Elen33. Enlightened Media. foodbytes. Geo-grafika. gulchuk. Ilyarexi. iquazu. jessmine. karandaev. Kovaleva Katerina. kungverylucky. Madlen. margo555. Maridav. maxsol. Morganka. Noregret. Olga Miltsova. Phanuwat Nandee. photooasis. Pincarel. Rudchenko Liliia. sarahdoow. sattva_ art. Scis65. videowokart. sierpniowka. sommai. sonyakamoz. stargatechris. Stargirl. Subbotina Anna. Suljo. EuToch. thisboy. Tiplyashin Anatoly. tpzijl. Valentina R. Valentina R. MayaMo. Viktar Malyshchyts. vrstudio. wollertz. yasonya. Yastremska. Courtesy www.bigstockphoto.com
All other photographs by C. Nathan Pulley Photography

Library of Congress Control Number: 2015953501

Ivory Soap is a trademark of Proctor and Gamble soaps.
Lipton Tea is a trademark of CONOPCO, INC.
Starbucks is a trademark of STARBUCKS.
Coca Cola is a trademark of the Coca Cola Company.
RR ROCKSTAR ENERGY DRINK trademark by Weiner, Russell G. in Las Vegas, NV, 89126.
Luzianne Coffee is a trademark of Reily Foods Company.

Type set in Avenir Next

ISBN: 978-0-7643-4954-6

Printed in China

Published by Schiffer Publishing, Ltd.
4880 Lower Valley Road
Atglen, PA 19310
Phone: (610) 593-1777; Fax: (610) 593-2002
E-mail: Info@schifferbooks.com

For our complete selection of fine books on this and related subjects, please visit our website at www.schifferbooks.com. You may also write for a free catalog.

This book may be purchased from the publisher. Please try your bookstore first. We are always looking for people to write books on new and related subjects. If you have an idea for a book, please contact us at proposals@schifferbooks.com.

Schiffer Publishing's titles are available at special discounts for bulk purchases for sales promotions or premiums. Special editions, including personalized covers, corporate imprints, and excerpts can be created in large quantities for special needs. For more information, contact the publisher.

Dedication

To my spiritual daughter, Sara Martinelli, a true tea master from whom I have learned so much and with whom I have enjoyed many a delicious cup of tea. Thank you for your insights, your encouragement, and your love.

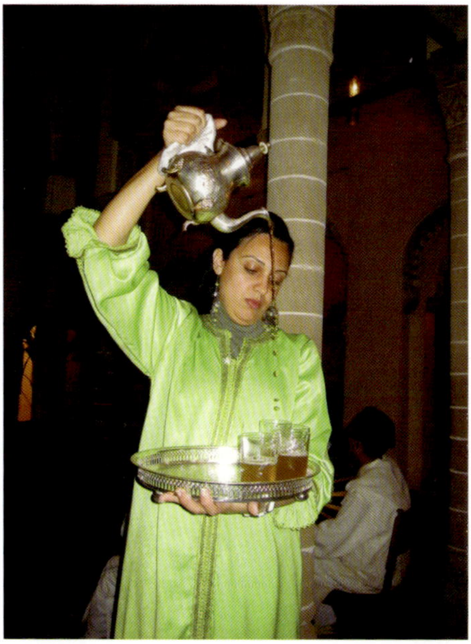

Moroccan Mint Tea. Served in Morocco from an Ibrik with a Flourish. *Photo courtesy of Sara Martinelli.*

CONTENTS

Part II

Part III

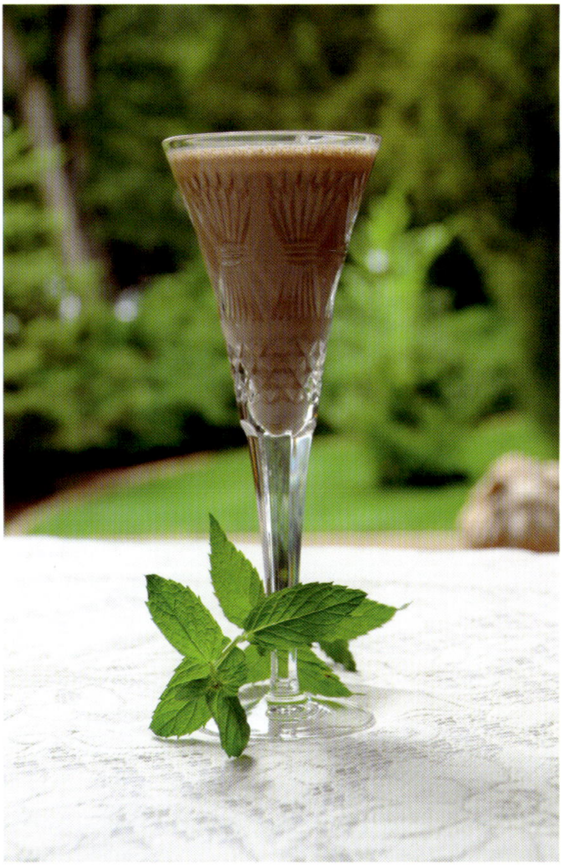

Luck o' the Irish Chocolate Mint Shake.
(Recipe on page 114.)

Acknowledgments

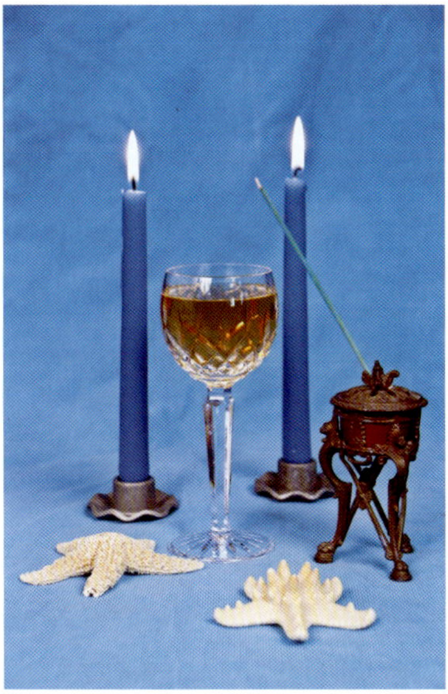

Apple Juice Meditation. Photo shows suggested altar setup.

I wish to thank my longtime friend Shauna Sandstead Corona for all the delicious *aguas frescas* recipes she has shared, and for her understanding of the mysteries of Mexican herbalism. Also to my good friend, Pocha (Flor) Crawford, for her many thoughtful insights into Peruvian and Latino culture and for introducing me to *Chicha Morada* and the delights of Peruvian cuisine. Many thanks to Sue Nash, friend, fellow writer, and consummate master of the English language, for her perspicacious comments and peerless knowledge of proper punctuation as well as her encouragement in my writing endeavors. Her suggestions were invaluable. A shout out goes also to Mike Smith and the staff of The Trident Bookstore and Café in Boulder, Colorado, who graciously provided some beautiful potions and allowed us to photograph them at their charming café. And this book would not be what it is without the creative eye and expertise of photographer Nathan Pulley. Thank you for your attention to detail, patience, dedication, and commitment to work on this project and for the splendid photos of my creations. Thanks, too, to my editor Dinah Roseberry, who tirelessly worked to help shape the manuscript. Lastly, and as always, I am indebted to my husband John O. Dow, my first reader and unflagging advocate of my literary pursuits, for his love, enthusiasm, inspiration, and faith in me and my endeavors over the years.

Part I

INTRODUCTION

You are here to learn the subtle science and exact art of potion-crafting...(and) understand the beauty of the softly simmering cauldron with its shimmering fumes, the delicate power of liquids that creep through human veins, bewitching the mind, ensnaring the senses....
–J. K. Rowling (b. 1965)
Author, Harry Potter and the Sorcerer's Stone

It's no coincidence that in *Harry Potter*, the popular children's fiction series, the most formidable teacher at Hogwarts Academy of Magic is the potions master. Belief in the capacity of potions to procure love, money, and success, protect and heal, and even wreak havoc and death, has been ingrained in the human psyche over the centuries through the retelling of myths and legends.

We all were raised on fairy tales from our different cultures. As a child, I adored the pretty princess in *Sleeping Beauty* who, after quaffing a sleeping draught, fell into a trance and was condemned to remain in a state of suspended animation until awakened by a kiss from a handsome prince. After reading *Alice in Wonderland*, I spent months wandering around the park near our home searching for a rabbit hole to climb down. Surely I would find a "Drink Me" draught to enable me to squeeze through the doorway to Wonderland.

Legendary tales of potions spill over into the adult psyche, too. Who can forget the bubbling witches' cauldron in *Macbeth*? Or the '60s pop song "Love Potion Number 9" that got an entire generation of "Flower Children" movin' and groovin'? Not to mention the scores of victims in murder mysteries who invariably make the very unwise decision to accept that poisoned cocktail or cup of coffee.

You don't have to be a fairy princess, a witch in a kids' movie, or a mystery lover to take pleasure in the enchantments of potions. Undoubtedly you have been drinking these brews all of your life without realizing it. When, as a child, you caught a cough, your mother probably made you swallow a syrupy concoction. This type of medicinal potion is known as an electuary. Perhaps this morning you breakfasted on a glass of orange juice because you believe its high vitamin C content starts your day out right. Maybe you also sipped hot milk or chamomile tea last night to help you fall asleep. These healthy beverages represent another aspect of the contemporary belief in the power of magical drinks.

At one time or another, you may have consumed a potion for reasons other than better health. For example, the ritual toast made with champagne, wine, or fruit juice to celebrate a special occasion, such as a wedding, anniversary, or birthday, shows a common social use of potions. In our household, I always knew the holidays were coming because my father brought home a bottle of Mogen David. Everyone, except my great-aunt, was not especially fond of this very sweet wine. It was the only alcoholic beverage Auntie would touch, and only then to celebrate the day. Even I was given a shot glassful so the entire family could participate in the toast.

The wine or grape juice taken at Communion in Christian churches and consumed by Jews at Passover shows a ritualistic spiritual use of liquids in religion. The Quechua and Aymará Indians of Peru, Ecuador, and Bolivia, as well as practitioners of Brazilian magical religions, Voodun, and Wicca imbibe wine, liquor, herbal infusions, and/or fruit juice potions at many of their ceremonies as libations to honor their deities. These are just a few examples of how potions permeate many aspects of our lives in contemporary times.

What's in a Potion?

Water is H2O, hydrogen two parts, oxygen one. But there is also a third thing that makes water and nobody knows what that is.
–D. H. Lawrence (1885–1930)
Author, Pansies, 1929.

What Lawrence says about water can apply to potions. A potion is any liquid you drink or give somebody else to consume because you have faith that it will produce a special effect. Belief comprises the third ineffable ingredient that separates potions from other drinks.

This definition excludes the favorite soda you guzzle along with Friday night's pizza while streaming DVDs because you probably don't believe it will produce any special effect on your body, except perhaps adding an extra pound or two to your frame. It also eliminates the ritual of roasting, carving, and eating the Thanksgiving turkey because turkey is a solid food. Most potions are designed to attract spiritual energy in the form of protection, strength, better health, and the universal love that flows from God, the deities, or the cosmos, according to each person's faith.

Whether the potions you create and consume actually are effective has a lot to do with your attitude. Keeping an open mind toward the experience and accepting that a potion has the potential to help make changes in your spiritual, mental, emotional, and physical body takes you halfway to success. The concept isn't hard to digest when you consider that sometimes you drink medicine to get well or sip fruit juices to stay in tip-top condition. Of course the potion's ingredients have a lot to do with its effectiveness, too.

When I lived in Rio de Janeiro, I couldn't help but notice the scores of hole-in-the-wall open-air bistros in every neighborhood that sold fruit juice concoctions. Ripe oranges, pineapples, avocados, mysterious-looking melons, varieties of nuts, and colorful fruits I'd never seen before, overflowed wire baskets swinging gaily from the rafters in the soft, tropical breeze. A customer could buy freshly squeezed juices in any combination, as well as drinks that the rest of us have come to know as smoothies. (Some recipes for them follow later). Brazilians call these places *Vitaminas* bars because they believe that consuming one of these vitamin-rich potions every day will keep illness at bay. Whether it is the ingredients, belief in the power of vitamins, or a combination of both, *Vitaminas* seem to work for Brazilians in the same way healthy smoothies assist us.

The kinds of drinkable potions are as limitless as the imagination. Examples include flavored and colored waters, teas, juices, smoothies, juleps, soups, sauces, syrups, vinegars, and even mysterious, medicinal-sounding concoctions such as philtres, elixirs, and electuaries.

Even liquids that are not drinkable like sprinkling waters, floor washes, massage oils, bath salts, and crystals that dissolve in water and help soften the skin, can be categorized as potions. Theoretically, perfumes are considered potions because they are comprised of liquids. You won't find any recipes for non-drinkable potions in this book. Their range is so vast it would take a separate book, or maybe even several volumes to do them justice. If you are interested in pursuing this angle of potion-crafting, I refer you to my books on the subject, *Witch's Brew* and *Green Magic* (both published by Schiffer Books).

What to Expect from This Book

In Part I, I open the faucet, so to speak, and introduce you to drinkable culinary potions that you can rustle up in your kitchen using ingredients you probably already have on hand or can find at the grocery or health food store. You will learn to formulate personalized recipes for health, love, money, career, beauty, self-realization, communications, domestic harmony, wisdom, and many other intentions. An array of potions including teas, coffees, and cocoa, colored waters–even beer–are described.

Part II offers scores of recipes to enhance various aspects of your life. If you have a flair for the culinary arts and/or are curious about the nutritional and psychological benefits of the ingredients you are using, you may want to move beyond my basic formulas to Part III. There you will find a full range of potion ingredients to fire your imagination. The list includes fruits and vegetables, along with their descriptions and beneficial components. Folklore associated with them that has been handed down through oral traditions over the ages is also mentioned.

The glossary of terms helps you understand health potion vocabulary. The bibliography of books, articles, and Internet resources is designed for those interested in further exploration of the topic.

Ethical Considerations

Before you launch on your journey into the marvelous world of potion-crafting, I want to address two important topics: the ethics of potion-crafting and the relationship between potions and alcohol.

When you start mixing potions for others, you need to ask yourself if it is morally correct to change a person's mental, emotional, spiritual, and physical state–especially without that person's knowledge and permission. Do you have the right to interfere in another human being's life? What could be the karmic consequences of your actions for yourself as well as for others?

The obvious answer to these questions is that you should only devise potions for yourself or for others with their knowledge and consent. Period. It is not fair to do something to or for someone without the individual's knowledge, no matter how noble your intentions.

Once you have the person's consent, you need to ask about food allergies. Think of all the people who are deathly allergic to the inoffensive looking little peanut. I have a friend who, if she munches even one spinach leaf, will immediately fall into anaphylactic shock. Don't assume you know a person's allergy history. Even your best friend or cousin whom you haven't seen for a while may have developed sudden sensitivities. As an added precaution, let the person know about all the ingredients you want to use to verify that it's okay with them. The old saw about an ounce of prevention really makes sense when it comes to potion-crafting.

Potions and Alcohol

Types of potions you won't find emphasized in this book are those that contain alcohol. In the first place, almost every fruit, vegetable, and herb that exists is attributed some kind of magical or medicinal value, so non-alcoholic substitutes are as effective as anything alcoholic if you are going for a magical effect.

Being a realist, I know that many people, including me, enjoy alcoholic beverages. A long tradition of alcohol consumption at special occasions—even if it's only my aunt's Mogen David wine—has provided a great deal of pleasure for people from cultures worldwide and over time. To my mind, moderation as in all things is the key to alcohol indulgence. So in this book, I occasionally offer recipes that include alcoholic ingredients. I even include a section on beer. But I also mention non-alcoholic alternatives.

I'll pause here to sip my tea potion concocted from fresh lemon balm leaves to help hone my communication skills, a pinch of cinnamon to inspire me, and a slice of lemon on the side for added energy, and lift my china cup to you in a toast. May you succeed in creating all the potions your heart desires for pleasure and to further your well-being.

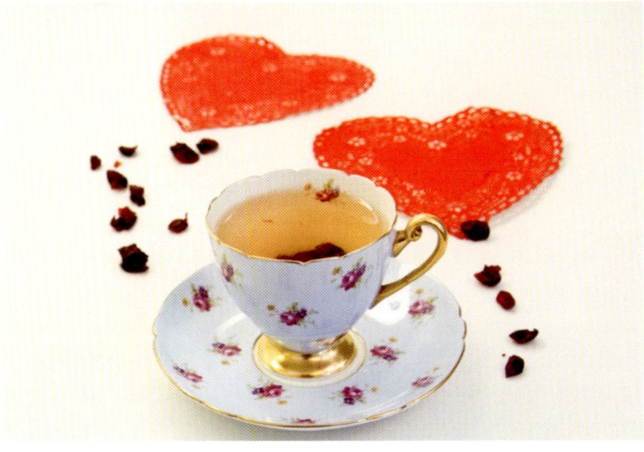

Valentine's Day White Peony Tea.
(Recipe on page 43.)

Chapter 1

WATERS OF LIFE AND THE POTION CRAFTER'S KITCHEN

Be praised, My Lord, through Sister Water;
She is very useful, and humble, and precious, and pure.
–Francis of Assisi (1181-1226)
Saint, Canticle of the Sun, circa 1225

Anybody who wants to create potions should first understand something of the magic of water. Not only does water cover more than seventy percent of the earth's surface, it comprises the major ingredient of many potions. It makes sense to learn something about its characteristics and apply its virtues to concoct yummy, wholesome drinks that just might affect deep levels of your consciousness as well. The notion that water can help make changes in consciousness may be a bit hard to swallow, so let me offer an explanation.

Water is one of the four primary elements that ancient cultures believed engendered life. Primitive people reasoned that since our physical bodies are mostly composed of water, all living beings emerged from a primordial ocean, the source of life. Our ancestors also observed that water dissolves and disseminates the solid, nutritional chemicals of earth into a liquid state so that the human organism can readily absorb and synthesize them.

By the same reasoning, water was thought to possess the ability to dissolve physical, mental, emotional, and spiritual impurities and superfluities, and deposit them in the earth for transmutation. This life-sustaining substance was considered female in nature and was associated with traditional feminine traits such as fertility, creativity, compassion, and seduction.

Water is deemed to contain the power to transform inner consciousness: that is, thoughts, emotions, and spirit. This is how the ceremony of baptism got started. The ritual symbolizes rebirth on the inner levels of consciousness. In this sense, anyone who drinks a water-based potion–coffee, tea, juice, soup are a few examples–performs a kind of water magic.

Liquid Potions, the Five Senses, and Four Elements

The secret to the magic of potions lies in how potions use water and the other three elements to easily engage the five senses. The four primary elements of nature are Earth, Fire, Air, and Water. The pot bubbling over the fire's flame changes the raw materials harvested from the land into sustenance. Stirring the pot lets in air so that the ingredients combine in a compatible way instead of burning up. Patience, concentration, timing, and listening to your intuition–a faculty associated with the Water element–tell you just the right amount of earth products to include to whip up the most delicious and effective potions.

How the elements combine in a potion helps make these refreshments a joy to behold. Listening to the pot simmer on the stove alerts our taste buds. By the time the rich, cooking smells reach our noses, we are salivating. Tasting and feeling the textures of different ingredients as they glide over the tongue makes for an undeniably sensual experience.

Potions and Color

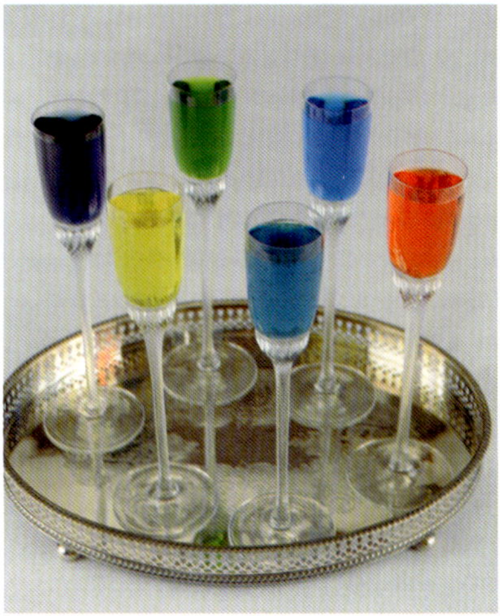
Photograph by C. Nathan Pulley Photography

Colored Waters.

The second piece of information to know before diving into the cupboards for the pots and blender is how to use color in your potions. The color of any food, including liquid potions, affects how people will react to it. Every herbal infusion, smoothie, soup, or sauce that you blend will have some color to it. Even one-ingredient potions, such as tea, come in a variety of colors from red to orange, green, yellow, or even brown. A blueberry smoothie is blue, cold cucumber soup is green, and so-on.

What the natural pigments of fruits and vegetable do, besides being visually appealing, is provide nutrition. The concept that everyone should eat a rainbow of colors daily from produce in order to maintain good health is a growing trend. For example, an orange mango *lassi*, a cold mango, yogurt, and milk treat served in many Indian restaurants, will energize you with vitamin C, soothe bronchial congestion, and even combat body odor. The chlorophyll in green-hued Gyokuro green tea will strengthen your teeth and bones and help prevent gum disease. The blueberries in the smoothie I mentioned above contain anthocyanin, a mighty antioxidant that can improve memory and reduce the risk of heart disease and stroke.

Along with the nutritional qualities of naturally colored food come remarkable psychological benefits. The therapeutic values of different hues have been acclaimed throughout history by diverse cultures such as Native Americans, Arabs, Celts, Central Asians, Chinese, Druids, Greeks, Persians, and Teutonic people. Ancient Egypt was celebrated for its color halls at Karnack and Thebes where research into color therapy and color healing was regularly performed.

Today, the study of color psychology and color therapy is a recognized discipline. Experts in the field, known as Chromotherapists, advocate the theory that disease is caused by imbalances in the physical, mental, emotional, and spiritual bodies. They theorize that these imbalances take place in the chakras, specific reservoirs of energy in the body. The function of a chakra is to absorb light and filter the colors needed to energize body, mind, and spirit. Sometimes the process of filtering ideal color frequencies is impeded by a blockage. The result is disharmony that may express itself as illness or disease. Chromotherapists restore balance by beaming appropriately colored lights on the distressed chakras. You can achieve a similar effect by drinking a colored potion.

Following are descriptions of colors to add to your potion-crafting palette. Included are symbolic meanings and some health benefits to be derived from

Depending on the other ingredients, pureed figs will turn a potion brown. So will peanut butter. Some of the darker mushrooms will do the same thing. And, of course, there are the classic potion ingredients cocoa and coffee. I discuss their many health benefits in later chapters.

White/Cream: I admit it isn't easy to create a completely white-colored potion. Usually it ends up looking cream-colored, unless all you use is milk, coconut milk, or egg whites. No matter! In color healing, this hue and all its creamy gradations stand for physical and spiritual cleansing, clairvoyance, healing, enlightenment, and clairvoyance. The whitish color comes from the chemical constituent anthoxanthin, which helps lower cholesterol and blood pressure. Popular whitish potion ingredients include banana, coconut, potato, and ginger.

Simple Color Recipes

If you yearn to reap the psychological benefits of drinking colored potions, but don't have the time or inclination to go to all the fuss of mixing ingredients in a blender, you can reap colorful rewards simply by adding a drop or two of food coloring to an eight-ounce glass of spring water. (Bottled spring water is readily available at the supermarket.) Most food coloring on the grocery shelf is blue, red, green, or yellow, and packaged in little boxes that contain all four colors.

- To make purple, mix one drop each of blue and red.
- To make orange, mix one drop of red with two of yellow.
- Red and green turn a potion brown.

If you want to go hog wild with shades of color, the guide on the package says to mix four blue and one green for turquoise, three yellow and one green for lime, four green and one yellow for pistachio, one red and two yellow for peach, and three red and two yellow for salmon. The photo on page 13 of this section shows the results of some of my efforts.

Color Your Potions Naturally

Perhaps you are sensitive to food coloring, or know somebody afflicted with ADD or ADHD, for whom food coloring may aggravate their symptoms. You can still enjoy colored waters because several companies now supply natural food coloring for drinks. The available hues may not be many and sometimes, especially when the coloring is an emulsion, they may turn the water the correct color, but a bit cloudy-looking. However, new water-soluble colors created from natural foods such as purple carrot, hibiscus, turmeric, grape skins, annatto seeds, paprika, and butterfly peas are currently being developed.

To purchase natural food coloring, check out a natural grocery store such as Whole Foods or Alfalfa's. You can also order these dyes online from companies like Seelect Inc. (www.seelecttea.com) and Wild Emulsions (www.wildflavors.com). If you're inclined to make your own, you can boil your own fruits and vegetables. Use the water that leaches out as a soup base and derive some physical health benefits in the bargain. Beets and asparagus are good examples.

Serves 2-4 (depending on cup size)

Just for Fun

GLOWING GELATIN TONIC WATER

Natural foods purists may frown upon the following recipe. I think it's so entertaining, I can't help but include it here. Most people realize that tonic water contains quinine, an ingredient of gin and tonic, and a chemical that has been prescribed to ward off the effects of malaria. What you may not know is that quinine glows bright blue when exposed to black light. Unfortunately (or fortunately, if you like the taste), quinine has a distinctive bitter flavor. To overcome some of the bitterness and still get the glow, follow this recipe:

Ingredients

- 1 cup water
- 1 3-ounce package flavored gelatin, any color. (You may substitute the sugar-free kind if you don't want the sugar.)
- 1 cup tonic water
- Glass mugs or cups
- 1 black light

Directions

Begin by bringing water to a boil. Dissolve gelatin in boiling water, and then add tonic water. Bring the mixture to a boil again. Pour into clear mugs and serve immediately under a black light.

If you wish, you can pour the mixture into four gelatin molds and let them set in the refrigerator. Serve like a regular gelatin dessert under a black light. You'll end up with a solid product that won't be an actual liquid potion, but you'll have a cool novelty to wow your friends.

Note: This recipe is for adults only as most children probably won't like the taste.

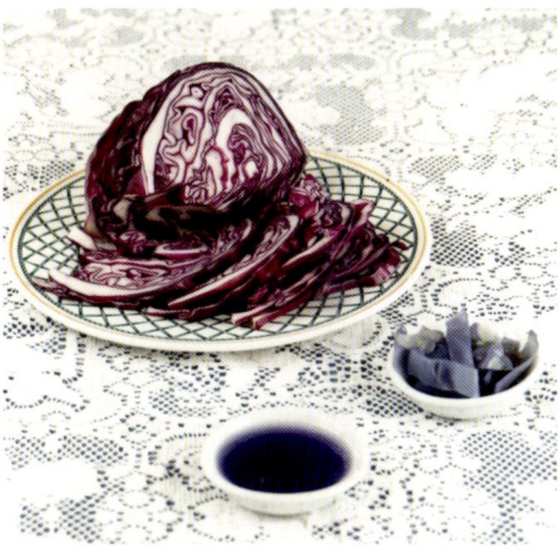

Photograph by C. Nathan Pulley Photography

Red Cabbage Water. Photo shows how simmering red cabbage in tap water shows the pH of the water. In this case, the pH level is neutral.

Red Cabbage and Your Water's pH

Before I leave the subject of potions and color, I'd like to add this tidbit. You can learn the pH of your water with red cabbage water by following these steps.

1. Cut a head into small pieces, place in a pot, and fill with tap water.
2. Simmer until the water colors.
   If the pH is neutral, the water will turn purple; if acidic, it will look red.
3. The water will be green if it is basic.

Note: You can do the same thing with blackberries, red onions, or hibiscus flowers.

Now that you've digested some of the theory behind potion-crafting, let's move on to the nitty-gritty of concoction.

Chapter 2

POTION-CRAFTING PRELIMINARIES

Your Sacred Space

Your sacred space is where you can find yourself again and again.
–Joseph Campbell (1904-87)
American mythologist, writer, and lecturer

Before you start conjuring potions, I suggest you clear the sacred space where you will prepare most of your formulas. I'm talking about your kitchen. Perhaps you never thought about this space in terms of the sacred, but I assure you, kitchens are more than convenient rooms to quickly heat and inhale meals. In bygone days, they served as centers of domestic activity. The entire family gathered around the hearth to dine, hash over the day's events, and sometimes spin yarns late into the night. Often the warmest room in the house, this space doubled as a nursery, and at times even a bedroom and schoolroom. In Feng Shui, the Chinese art of living well by creating balance in your environment, the kitchen represents the heart of the household, the center of its vital force.

The person in charge of the home has always held undisputed reign over the place where food is prepared. All sorts of superstitions have evolved around cooks and kitchens. Following is a variation of the adage, "Too many cooks spoil the broth." It is taken from my own experience and serves to underscore my point about cooks and the sacred nature of kitchens.

When I lived at the home of an elderly gentleman in Scotland, I had many occasions to prepare dinner. This tradition-bound man would permit no one in the kitchen with me while I worked–not even a helper. He told me that when he was a child, his mother laid down this household rule. She claimed that comings and goings diverted her attention and hindered her intuitive ability to combine just the right ingredients. Any disturbance whatsoever might cause her to spoil an entire meal–an unthinkable horror for the penny-wise Scots. To me, this attitude shows ultimate respect for a person's private precinct, as well as the esteem in which the kitchen and the cook are held.

In my own home, I'd say "fat chance" to the opportunity of ever getting enough peace and quiet to prepare a meal without interference, let alone a potion. Everything, including the proverbial kitchen sink, ends up parked in this room. As I write at my kitchen table I'm gazing at a pair of snow skis propped against a wall, Halloween costumes carelessly thrown over a chair, a power drill decorating the counter, and twenty pounds of kitty litter blocking the entryway. The refrigerator, to put it kindly, stores many fond memories of past meals—some of those meals from the very distant past. The front of this anthropological artifact is plastered with coupons, family photos, and postcards from friends who've traveled to exotic places I'll never see. Nevertheless, my kitchen is a warm, cozy room, often filled with friends and loved ones engaged in lively discussions.

At night after the house quiets down, I sit at the table of my "Queendom" in blissful solitude. Slowly, I sip a relaxing potion of chamomile tea with hints of hops and vanilla and contemplate the day's events and sometimes even the meaning of life.

If my kitchen sounds like yours, before you get down to serious potion-crafting you'll want to transform it into a sacred space—or at least a sacred space in progress. I say "in progress" because it probably goes through various incarnations from clean and reverent to chaotic and just plain dirty, often over the space of a day. Whenever you feel the need to reclaim the sacred, here's what to do:

1. Your first step is to tidy up really well. Sweep the floor with a broom. In many cultures, brooms stand for spiritual cleansing.
2. Next, wash the floor with vinegar and water. In the Voodun religion, the power of vinegar to physically cleanse an environment is assumed, by analogy, to imbue it with the power to purify spiritually. Temple floors are scrubbed vigorously with vinegar and water to chase away evil spirits and impure thoughts.
3. If, after exerting all that elbow grease, you still feel enthusiastic about cleaning, sprinkle on the floor a mixture of water into which you have dissolved a few salt granules.
4. Repeat the procedure with cabinets, stove, sink, table, and chairs to further purify the space. These measures, however, are not necessary.
5. Weather permitting, open a window or door and, if possible, freshen the room with flowers. Hang fragrant herbs to dry in the high space over the sink well away from the stove. Burn a stick of culinary incense like cinnamon, vanilla, or clove, and light candles to create a positive environment.
6. For a special touch, place an open bowl of spicy potpourri on the counter and play soothing music while you work. You can even try a trick a real-estate friend once shared. She said that when your house goes on the market, you should throw a few fresh orange, lemon, or tangerine peels into the disposal and grind them up. It will eliminate cooking odors, give the kitchen a sweet, citrusy scent, and lend a cozy feel to the place.

Apple Juice Meditation Treat

You've worked so hard scrubbing and polishing, and your kitchen is sparkling like a sunny spring morning. I think you deserve a treat, don't you? Time to kick back at your uncluttered, gleaming kitchen table and enjoy the fruits of your labor by quaffing a simple but mighty apple juice potion. The ancient Celts believed that apples impart great knowledge and wisdom, so this juice makes an ideal potion for relaxation and contemplation.

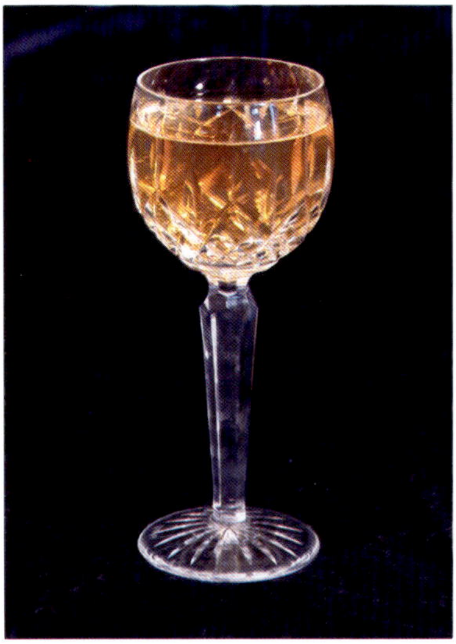

Photograph by C. Nathan Pulley Photography

Apple Juice Meditation Treat.

The following meditation is designed to enhance your enjoyment and appreciation of potion ingredients in general and help you become a first-rate potions expert. Drink it any time you want to dust away the cobwebs from your mind, solve problems, open your inner life to creativity and spirituality, and–according to my husband–immensely improve your humor.

For this exercise you'll need:

2 blue tapers (as you recall, this hue fosters harmony)

Candle holders

a stick of cinnamon incense (for mental stimulation)

An incense burner, matches

A clear glass filled with cold apple juice.

For once, I recommend you don't use organic apple juice unless it is very transparent because organic juice can look muddy in the glass. You want a clear liquid to mirror a calm, untroubled mind.

Place the glass of juice in front of you on the table and the candles on either side. Put the incense burner in a convenient spot where you won't breathe in the smoke directly. Light the tapers and incense.

Take a comfortable seat in an upright chair in front of the glass and fix your gaze on the cup. Immerse your thoughts in the amber liquid. Imagine that the wetness and freshness of the juice is pouring over you like limpid water from a pristine sea. Don't drink the juice yet, but mentally taste its tangy sweetness.

After a few moments, visualize yourself diving deep into the liquid, swimming effortlessly like a fish along the ocean floor. As you slide through this fathomless, silent sea, take a look at the exquisite marine life that has materialized around you–starfish gleaming on the ocean floor, brilliantly colored seaweed swaying in the currents, exotic fish swimming soundlessly through the depths.

Eventually you arrive at a subterranean castle fashioned from pink coral, barnacles, shells, and bits of netting. A beautiful mermaid with flowing, flaxen hair and sapphire eyes appears in the doorway and beckons. Swim to her and ask her to guide you on the path to inner knowledge. Listen to her message.

After a few minutes' communion with the enchanting mermaid, thank her for her wise counsel. Then turn and glide out of the sea castle and back home. Slowly float to the surface of the water as if emerging from a deep pool.

Presto! You're back in your kitchen once more. Sip the apple juice and savor its piquant, refreshing sweetness. What bliss!

Chapter 3

POTION-CRAFTING TOOLS

Tools of the Trade

As a carpenter knows what to do with his hammer and saw and a pro golfer understands her clubs, if you are going to get serious about potion-crafting, you'll need to familiarize yourself with the tools of your trade.

Potion craftsmanship is an unpretentious but prodigious art that always has and continues to be performed by cooks every day. Its magic gains strength from constant use of common tools and ingredients. If I were a betting person, I'd wager you already have most of the tools you require squirreled away in your kitchen drawers and cabinets. What you might not realize is that each of these implements is associated with one of the elements of nature I talked about earlier. Following are some basic tools and their elemental correspondences.

Air Tools

I've already mentioned using a broom to purify the kitchen. Because brooms make sweeping motions, this tool is linked to the element Air. Other tools associated with Air include the blender, juicer, beater, spoon, and fork. These implements facilitate the free intermingling of ingredients in a container and stir up their energy. The fork, besides accomplishing this task, penetrates the ingredients in the same way perceptions penetrate the mind.

The knife is another Air tool that trims away excess with its sharpness. By analogy, it cuts away all that is unnecessary or obstructive for making your potion succeed. Even the kitchen window represents an instrument of Air because it invites the fresh breeze to stimulate and vitalize your brews.

Fire Tools

The stove, microwave, and other heating implements relate to Fire because they transmute many of the raw ingredients into potions through the medium of heat. The soups, sauces, teas, coffees, and cocoa recipes in this book all rely on heat for preparation.

Earth Tools

As to the Earth element, the ingredients themselves are products of the soil, and therefore, earthy in nature. The cupboards, pantry, and drawers that store and keep safe the ingredients and tools are also associated with this element.

Water Tools

The pot, cauldron, kettle, glass, and cup all connect to Water because these containers hold liquids. The sink and dishwasher, too, fall under the guardianship of this element. So, too, does the funnel, filter, and infuser because they trap impediments to ease the flow of the liquid.

Cup Symbolism

Because you'll drink most of your potions from cups, glasses, and bowls, I'd like to spend a few minutes describing the symbolism of this important tool.

In some cultures it is believed that a person's soul is contained in the cup because these vessels are thought to contain the essence of life. Some concepts associated with the cup, or chalice, as it is sometimes called, include love, fertility, understanding, ecstasy, and communication.

Why communication? Because receptacles conduct our words through the sense of hearing. To understand this idea, hold against your ear a conch shell, which is a type of container, and listen to the tide. In the Bible, Gabriel, the Archangel of Water, blows a trumpet, which is a variation of a conch shell. He is considered the messenger or medium between human and divine intelligence. The trumpet becomes a horn. In turn, the horn can be interpreted to represent a phallic horn inside of which lies the cup, a female symbol of fertility. Gabriel becomes the life-bearer who, driven by the power of Love, turns force into form.

Cups also give form to our thoughts and words because without them, whatever we put into the cup would disintegrate and flow away. You can never empty a cup because something will always fill it, even if it is simply air. The contents of the cup are always changing because it is constantly being emptied or filled. When you drink the liquid, you transfer its form, that is, the contents, from one receptacle (the cup) to another (your body). In this way, you execute a transformation. Whatever you desire the cup to contain will flow along with the liquid inside you to help make changes on inner levels of your being. This is true magic and so easy!

All of this awesome talk about cups doesn't mean you should run out and buy expensive china or crystal to hold your potions. What you use daily will work just fine. It's the mindfulness and respect you apply when you use your cup or any of your other tools or ingredients that make potion magic work.

Having said that, you might want to purify one special glass or cup to use exclusively for potion artistry. When you first acquire your vessel, wash it thoroughly with a mild detergent such as Ivory Soap™. This cleansing dissolves any negativity that may be left clinging to it from the manufacturer or from someone who has handled it. Add a boost of power by again immersing it in a mixture of a few grains of salt dissolved in water. Repeat this process every time you use the container for potions.

Word of Advice

Now that you've identified the tools you're going to need and understand how you can make them work for you on a spiritual level, all that's left is to gather together your ingredients and get started. When it comes to ingredients, here's my two cents worth of advice:

Before you begin, make sure you have placed on the kitchen counter everything you'll need to build your potion. Nothing thwarts inspiration, concentration, and visualization more than to have to run to the store for a missing item. This is the voice of experience talking!

Mexican *Aguas Frescas*

In succeeding chapters, you'll learn to prepare straightforward liquid potions such as teas, coffees, smoothies, juices, soups, and sauces. To fortify you for the journey, I'll end this chapter with two of my favorite potion recipes for Mexican *aguas frescas*, fresh, flavored waters.

In Mexico, these waters predate sodas and continue to be popular today. *Aguas frescas* take advantage of the amazing variety of fruits and vegetables available in that country year round. Typically, they are drunk at mealtime and so are associated with peace, harmony, and contentment in the home. *Aguas frescas* are among my favorite potions because I treasure happy memories of drinking them when I lived in Mexico City as a teen. These particular recipes were given to me by my good friend, Shauna Sanstead-Corona, an expert on Mexican cuisine, who has lived in Mexico for many years.

Serves 4-6

Agua de Limón—LIME WATER

By far, the most popular agua fresca in Mexico is made from limes. People drink lime water on a daily basis. It is similar to limeade, but tastes lighter and less sweet. Since the resulting potion is clear green in color, you can drink it to achieve spiritual healing and draw peace and harmony to the home.

Ingredients

- ⅛ – ¼ cup sugar
- 1 quart water
- 5 small limes

Directions

Dissolve the sugar in the water. Then squeeze 5 small limes into the mixture. Stir and serve. *Salud!*

Serves 4-6

Agua de Jamaica— HIBISCUS WATER

Photograph by C. Nathan Pulley Photography

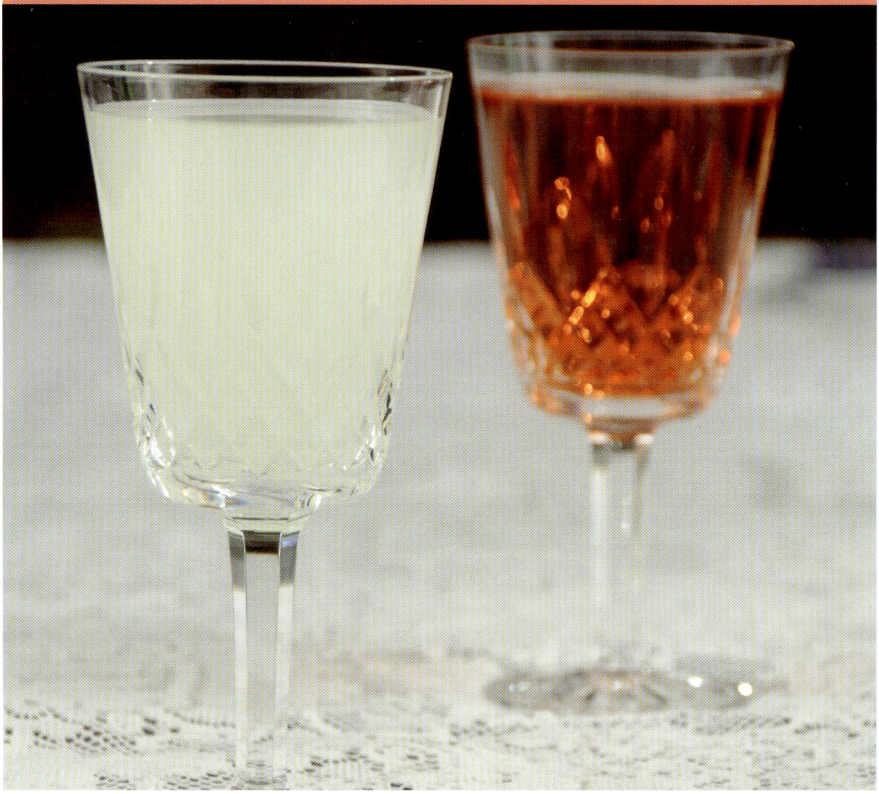

Ingredients

1 pound dried hibiscus flowers

1 quart water

Sugar, honey, or stevia to taste

Directions

Rinse the flowers well, cover them with water, and boil. When the flowers look pale, drain the water through a sieve into another pot. If the water doesn't appear very red, add more flowers and boil again. Let the water sit until the sediment from the flowers settles to the bottom. Drain off the water again. Add around a cup of this mixture to a quart of water. Sweeten to taste while the water is still warm and stir. Refrigerate and serve. Drink this potion to increase vigor, passion, and willpower.

Image: Agua de Jamaica (Mexican Hibiscus Water) and Agua de Limón (Mexican Lime Water).

Chapter 4

JUST YOUR CUP OF TEA

In this chapter you will find a lot of information about tea. This is because tea and herbal teas are my favorite "go-to" ingredients for potion-crafting. I'll define tea, tell you some of its history, and demystify different types of tea. You'll also learn about how tea can be good for your health and discover some current tea trends. I end the chapter with three tea potions I think you're bound to enjoy.

Tea is the second most popular drink in the world, ranking just behind water. In the US, coffee is more popular than tea (which just may have something to do with the Boston Tea Party and the American Revolution!). Even so, tea drinking is becoming more widespread every day.

Part of the enchantment may derive from the perception that tea—particularly specialty tea—is an affordable luxury. Tea experts evaluate tea in very much the same way wine buffs appraise wine.

Besides serving and drinking gourmet teas, the serious connoisseur can spend a fortune in order to acquire tea-related items such as antique teapots and tea sets. The desire to take tea in an elegant setting is one reason hotels that serve afternoon tea are now commonly found in most major metropolitan areas. It is also why the number of restaurants offering superior quality teas has been increasing.

Another powerful motivation has to do with tea's acclaimed health benefits. Gen-Xers and baby boomers struggling to preserve their youth and well-being as well as health gurus like Dr. Oz are singing tea's praises.

The idea of taking tea also evokes nostalgic feelings for times gone by. It reminds people of a more tranquil era when life moved at a slower, relaxed pace that allowed time to socialize with friends and family in a cozy environment. These tea lovers cast their minds back to the genteel epoch immortalized in novels by the likes of Jane Austen and Lewis Carroll, where tea plays a predominant role. They seek to recapture the elegance and comforts of the era by indulging in tea and sometimes dressing up in Victorian attire. In this way, tea does more than nourish the body; it feeds the soul.

Something I discovered during my research for this chapter is that many current trends are not really new at all; they simply have been reinvented. For instance, one of the latest "discoveries," white tea, has always been around, but its virtues as a healthy drink have not been well known in the West until recently. Similarly, the fact that green tea can be drunk to help cure common aches and pains was a main topic of the first book on tea, written in China in 780 CE. Tea liqueurs fashionable with the young martini-and-margarita set are basically permutations of the old English hot toddy, which combined tea and rum. Since tea has been around for so long, let's first travel back in time to learn about its evolution.

A Spoonful of Tea History

Five thousand years ago, Shen Nung, a Chinese emperor, was relaxing in a hammock in the Imperial Garden. A light breeze ruffled the surface of the water boiling in a pot set over a fire beneath a nearby Camellia tree. Leaves loosened from a branch and drifted into the hot water, releasing a heavenly fragrance that roused the sovereign and prompted him to taste the brew. Thus, as the legend goes, tea was discovered.

The Chinese called tea "The River of Jade" because, at first, they drank only unprocessed green leaves as a health potion that they considered of equal value to that precious mineral. Tea was not enjoyed as a beverage among all social classes until the Ming Dynasty (1368–1644 CE). The Japanese only learned about it after 1191 when a Buddhist monk returned from a trip to China with the seeds.

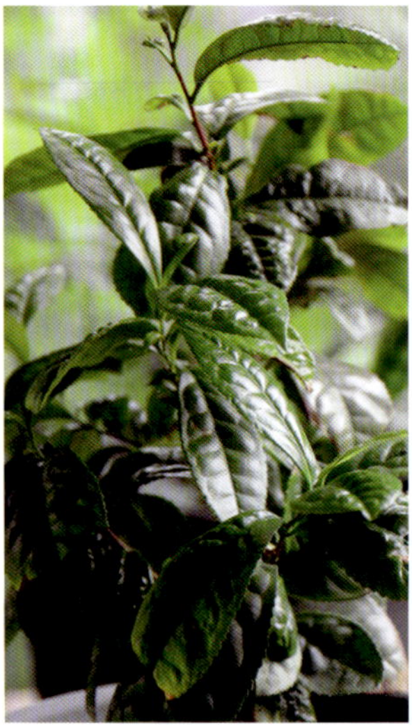

Photograph by C. Nathan Pulley Photography

Morwyn's Camellia sinensis Tea Plant.

The Japanese introduced tea to the West in the early 1600s, sending to the Netherlands a shipment of tea, which they touted as a medicinal potion. Catherine of Braganza, the Portuguese queen of Charles II of England, established the custom of taking tea in Britain because she believed it to be far healthier than alcohol. So rare and expensive was tea that well-to-do housewives kept it locked in tin or wooden caddies so servants would not be tempted to pilfer the precious commodity. Extravagant tea parties soon became fashionable in high society.

It seems, however, that you can't keep a good beverage limited to the privileged few. Through a variety of machinations, including stealing seeds and plants from the Chinese and smuggling tea around the world after high import tariffs were imposed, tea drinking eventually spread to all classes. With inventions such as cut and tear machines that quickly process leaves, serving tea iced as well as hot, and the convenience of teabags, the pleasures and benefits to be derived from tea eventually became readily and cheaply accessible to all.

What's Brewing in the Teapot?

All real tea, be it black, green, oolong, or white, come from the same kind of Camellia tree, whose name in Latin is *Camellia sinensis.* Other herbal drinks often referred to as herbal teas properly should be called "herbal infusions" or "tisanes." If you visit a tea garden, which is a plantation where tea is cultivated, you will see that the growers have pruned the trees to the size of a shrub to make picking the leaves easier.

To visit that tea garden you will probably have to journey to a high altitude, humid, equatorial region. The tea bush thrives in those areas, often on the shady side of a slope. Tea is grown in many countries around the world, including Japan, India, Sri Lanka, Kenya, Mozambique, Taiwan, Guatemala, Argentina, Papua/New Guinea, and even in such far-flung places as Australia and Cornwall, England. Today, the Chinese, who used to grow all of the world's tea, produce only around ten percent.

It might surprise you to know that some tea is cultivated right here in the US, if only in small quantities. Tea is harvested in South Carolina, Alabama, Hawaii, and Washington State. If you are strong-minded about buying American, check out American Classic Tea produced by The Bigelow Tea Company. You'll be in classy company, too, as this is the official tea of the White House. (As a gardening enthusiast, when I discovered this fact, I absolutely had to try growing my own tea bushes. Although I must constantly mist them in the dry climate where I live and bring them indoors during the cold winter months, I am the proud owner of two *camellia sinensis* bushes.)

Types of Tea

At the beginning of the last section, I mentioned four different types of tea. Although all come from the same bush, they don't grow like different kinds of fruit grafted on the same tree. The four types result, among other factors, from when and how much of the leaf is plucked. The different processing techniques play an important role, chiefly the length of time leaves are allowed to ferment before drying. This fermentation process, known as "oxidation," occurs after the leaves are spread on racks to wither. Then they either are cut and torn or twisted and rolled. This process breaks up the leaf cells and release the essential oils, which remain on the leaves. Oxidation also influences how much caffeine and how many tannins remain in the leaves. This, in turn, affects the taste.

White tea, which is a kind of green tea, is the least processed type. Only the unopened buds and first leaves to venture forth are picked. Green teas are also made from the unopened leaf buds and include the first two leaves. The leaves are then pan-fried or steamed, and quickly rolled and dried to limit oxidation. Both white and green teas tend to taste grassy.

I like to call the partially oxidized Oolongs "stealth teas" because this fine type is little known to the general public and barely marketed. It can be ferreted out at gourmet tea stores and, in my opinion, the hunt is well worth the trouble. Oolongs hail mainly from China and Taiwan and are the teas most often drunk during the traditional Gung Fu tea ceremony. These teas are withered and bruised to release the essential oils, and then partially oxidized, rolled, and dried. They can taste anywhere from peachy and melon-like to freshly green, rich, or woody.

Black teas, with which most of us are familiar, are fully oxidized teas, and therefore contain the most caffeine and tannins. These are full-bodied, stronger tasting teas. Depending on the kind of black tea, growers may pick more leaves and they may either roll or cut and tear them, often using a machine before drying or firing.

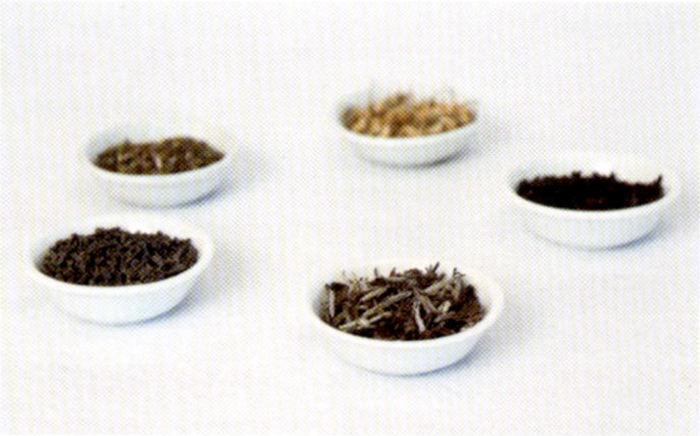

Photograph by C. Nathan Pulley Photography

Dry Teas. Photo shows Darjeeling, Gunpowder Green, White Peony, Chamomile, and Peppermint.

Blended and Scented Teas

Like a good Bordeaux, Chianti, Rioja, or Côtes-du-Rhône wine, tea can be blended or scented for a flavorful variation. Tea blends often combine two or more varieties. Ceylon teas often are selected for their superb flavor, Indian Assam for strength, and African varieties for color.

To create scented teas, manufacturers add full flower blossoms, fruit, peels, or herbs during the drying process. This imparts a delicate aroma and flavor. Arguably, the most popular scented tea is Earl Grey, whose piquant signature aroma comes from scenting black tea with bergamot mint leaves. Pouchang, a partially fermented, mild tasting tea produced in the Wenshan region of China and in Taiwan, is often used to offset the strong flavor of some of the harsher tasting green teas. Rose Pouchang, a tea scented with dried rose petals, is a delectable example. Those who frequent Chinese restaurants are probably familiar with jasmine tea, a standby served in such establishments. Some manufacturers use essential oils to scent teas. Always read the label to make sure the tea has been scented with true essences, not synthetics, as scents concocted in laboratories can be harmful if ingested.

One scented tea celebrated throughout the Middle East is called Moroccan Mint. This thirst quencher blends green tea with spearmint, peppermint, and wild mint leaves. By tradition, it is served with a flourish from a pot with a long spout, which you can see in the photo on page 3 of the Dedication.

Too Much Choice? Finding the Very Best Tea

Frankly, I don't believe a person can ever have too much choice when it comes to selecting tea. I do understand how the plentiful varieties available can be overwhelming, especially to the new tea consumer. Given the current tea craze, more are popping up on the market than dandelions in the spring garden. (Incidentally, dandelion leaf and root can be made into delicious herbal health potions). How to weed them out?

Tea Grades

One way to judge a tea is to pay attention to its grade. Usually it is printed in capital letters on the side of the package or can. Examples include: BOP (broken, large-leaf orange pekoe) and GFOP (golden colored young tips or buds plucked early in the season). An industry joke claims that the upscale grade of one Souchong, SFTGOFOP, really means "Far Too Good For Ordinary People."

In this complicated system different types of tea are assessed differently. Green and white teas are graded according to leaf age, style, and size with the best quality coming from lightly rolled, early buds and leaves. They often look clear to greenish-yellow in the cup so can be used to represent those hues in color healing. Oolongs have a wide range of flavors, scents, and colors and can be infused several times. They are ranked according to aroma (floral or fruity), taste, aftertaste, quality of the leaf, and whether or not they have been roasted. Black teas are graded according to leaf size and appearance. In your teacup, a black tea will look reddish-orange to reddish-brown–unless, of course, you over-brew it, in which case, it will look like mud! In potion-crafting, black tea is associated with good health and energy.

One useful term you might want to add to your vocabulary is "choppy." It refers to a tea lot that contains leaves of various sizes. Another descriptor, "tippy," refers to the abundance of downy white or yellow hairs that appear on the tips of the youngest leaves. Tippy tea is usually of superior quality.

Experts called tea tasters train to taste and grade teas at all stages of production, brokerage, and blending. In contemporary times, Noble "Toby" Fleming (he died in 2013), was one of the world's most famous tea tasters. He was apprenticed to Lipton Teas™ in 1938 and rose to become the arbiter of taste for the company, which is the biggest seller of tea in the US.

Every day at the Lipton laboratory in Englewood Cliffs, New Jersey, Fleming sipped tea from hundreds of china cups to evaluate which varieties to buy. Just like a wine-taster, he used a chrome-plated cuspidor to spit out the tea, then chewed on an apple to clear his palate. Fleming became one of the world's top twenty-five tea masters and trained many other professionals.

For detailed descriptions of tea grades, I refer you to www.mightyleaf.com or www.tealaden.com/teaweb/articles/art_grading_tea.

A Baker's Dozen of Fine Teas

Another way to decide which tea you might want to try is to read some descriptions. Too many wonderful teas exist to name all of my favorites, let alone all that are on the market, so I have had to make tough choices. Each one tastes fabulous on its own, and all combine successfully with other botanicals, milk, ice cream, even soups and sauces, to create first rate potions.

Since this is a cookbook, I will describe a baker's dozen of the most popular. The list includes black, oolong, green, and white teas.

ASSAM

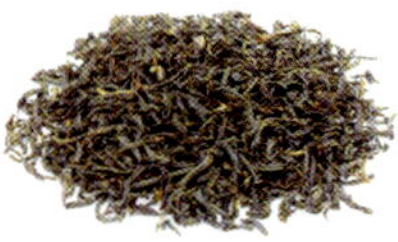

More black tea is cultivated in this Indian state than in any other region. Assam teas have a pleasant biscuit-like aroma and malty taste. If you go for Afternoon Tea at The Ritz Hotel in London, they will ask you if you prefer India or China tea, meaning Assam or Keemun. Recently I took Afternoon Tea at The Ritz in Manhattan and was pleased to learn that their menu offers a wide assortment of teas, including herbal infusions.

CEYLON

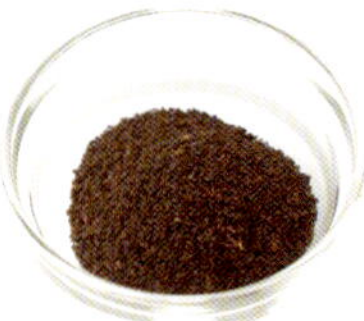

This black tea from Sri Lanka (formerly known as Ceylon, hence the name), supplies the base for many blends. Ceylon's flowery aroma and light aftertaste make it an ideal ingredient for many potions. Since the brewed tea looks bright orange in the teacup, it can represent this hue in color healing.

DARJEELING

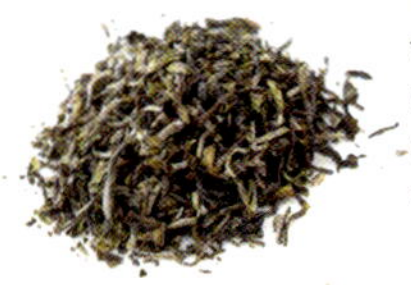

This exquisite black tea grown at high altitude in India's Himalayas enjoys the reputation as the "champagne of teas." Its taste is flowery and fresh with a hint of Muscatel. I find that Darjeeling's warm and spicy flavor makes an exceptional potion. In the cup the tea looks like liquid amber, and so can be used to represent orange, red, and brown in color healing.

DRAGONWELL

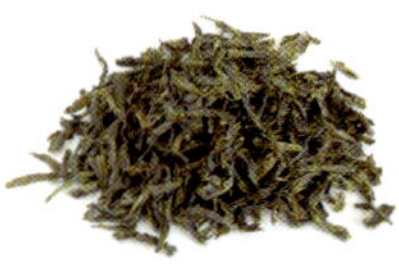

One of the earliest teas on record is this hand-tossed China green tea. The sweet but smooth flavor is an asset in many potions. The best of the six grades of Dragonwell is hand-tossed in special iron pans. In the cup, the liquid shimmers clear yellow, like the citrine gemstone and so can be used to represent the yellow hue in color healing.

EARL GREY

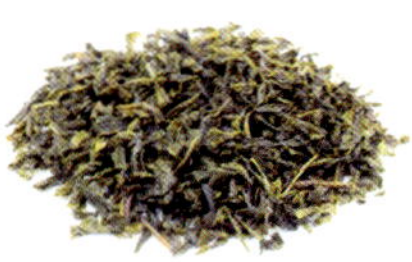

Jean-Luc Picard in *Star Trek, The Next Generation,* on ordering his favorite tea, once commented, "And whoever this 'Earl Grey' fellow is, I'd like to have a word with him!" Here is where the captain can be enlightened. It is said that a Chinese mandarin presented the secret formula to a British Prime Minister for having accomplished a successful diplomatic mission. Earl Grey blends China black and Darjeeling teas and is scented with citrusy oil of bergamot. Lady Grey, a popular variety, adds either lavender or Seville orange peel to the recipe.

FORMOSA OOLONG

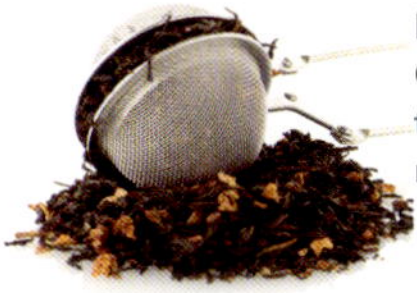

As its name indicates, this tea hails from Taiwan (formerly known as Formosa, which is Portuguese for "beautiful"). It blends partially oxidized China teas scented with peach blossoms to create an inviting liquor and toasty flavor. Herbalists recommend this reddish-brown colored oolong to mitigate symptoms of neurological diseases, such as Parkinson's.

GUNPOWDER

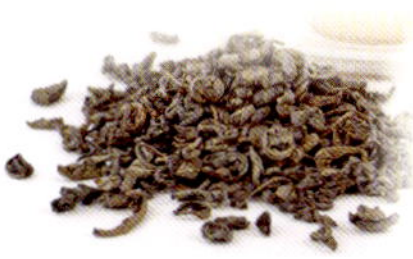

This green tea is named for the grayish-green color of the young leaves. The leaves are painstakingly rolled into little pearls (the Chinese call it *zucha*, Pearl Tea). The pearls also resemble gunpowder pellets, hence the name in English. Because the pearls are so tightly rolled, this type of tea keeps longer than other greens. The robust flavor with the lingering aftertaste of this fairly oxidized tea is similar to black tea. Gunpowder makes an excellent "green starter tea" for those not accustomed to the harsh or grassy taste of some green teas. The greenish-brown brew can represent these hues in color healing. When I perform tealeaf readings, I often use Gunpowder for single-question readings. As the pellets unfurl, they make a few, bold, easily interpretable images on the side of the cup.

JASMINE SILVER NEEDLES

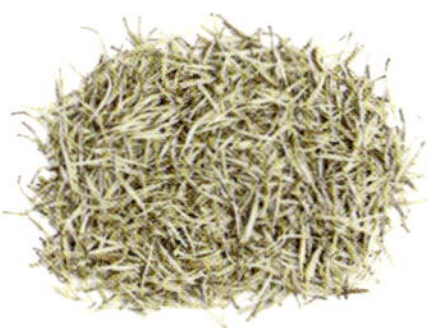

This China white tea is made from soft, downy buds and is lauded for its light, sweet taste. The buds are picked in the Fujian Province in April. After they dry in the soft sunlight, they are laid beneath a bed of fresh jasmine blossoms to soak up the aroma. Jasmine Silver Needles can represent the white hue in color healing. The tea makes a perfect choice for relaxation.

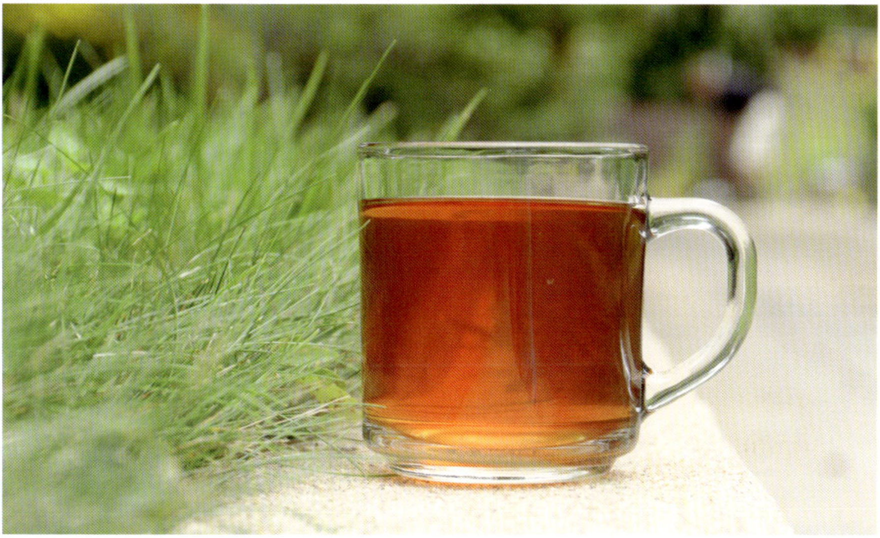

Photograph by C. Nathan Pulley Photography

Orange Pekoe Tea. Note the clarity of the orange tones.

MATCHA

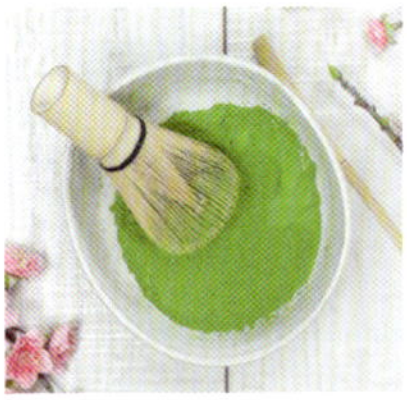

Those who frequent Japanese restaurants may be familiar with this tea as it flavors green ice cream. The whole-leaf tea is cultivated on the shady slopes of the Fuji region. The Japanese crush the leaves in a stone mill and use them in their celebrated tea ceremony. Because the powder dissolves easily in liquid, which turns a mellow green hue, Matcha tea makes a convenient ingredient for many kinds of potions. The green color encourages harmony and balance. Because the entire leaf is processed, this tea is loaded with nutrients and amino acids.

ORANGE PEKOE

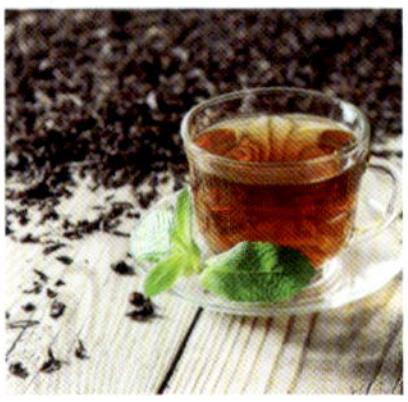

This fully oxidized, large-leaf black tea looks orange in the cup, but that is not how it got its name. When Orange Pekoe was first marketed in the West, it was touted as the preferred tea of the Royal Dutch House of Orange. Use it in orange-colored healing potions (see photo). This tea is grown mainly in Sri Lanka and southern India. Most readers may be familiar with Orange Pekoe (pronounced "peck-oh") because it is the tea used to fill Lipton teabags. The best ones taste fruity with a tangy aftertaste.

SENCHA

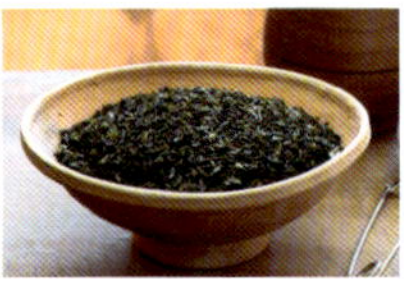

The Japanese drink this first-class fresh-tasting green tea daily in the same way many Americans imbibe Lipton's. While many teas prefer shaded growing conditions, Sencha is cultivated in the sun. Therefore, the leaf contains a hefty dose of antioxidants. In the cup, Sencha looks emerald green, and so can represent that hue in color healing.

TI KUAN YIN

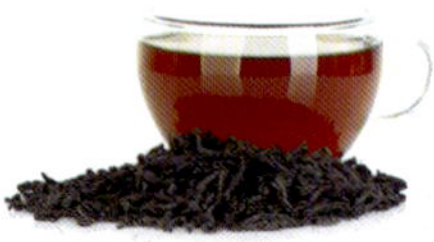

This rare oolong is named for the Chinese iron goddess of compassion and is arguably the most famous oolong of all. Legend has it that Buddhist monks trained monkeys to pick the delicate leaves and so, the tea is also called "Monkey Picked Oolong." The aroma of the pale golden liquor combines flowery sweetness with the rich greenness of the forest floor. The flavor is full-bodied and vegetal with slight floral notes. Ti Kuan Yin tea can be infused several times, and each infusion reveals a fresh complexity of flavor.

WHITE PEONY

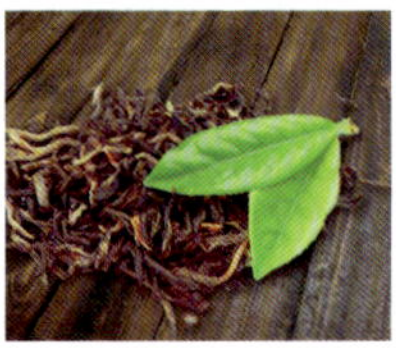

This mellow-tasting white tea is a choice variety. While its rival Silver Needles (described above) is made entirely of downy buds, White Peony includes one bud for every two leaves. This tea is known as an "easy tasting tea"; that is, it is mild and soothing on the palate. It tastes fresh and floral with underlying notes of malt and new mown hay. When the tightly rolled leaves unfurl in the cup they turn a brownish-green color and can be used to represent these hues in color healing. White Peony makes an excellent potion for grounding and centering. Some connoisseurs prefer to let this tea mature for a few years to lose all of the sharpness and increase the sweetness.

TEABAG TEA

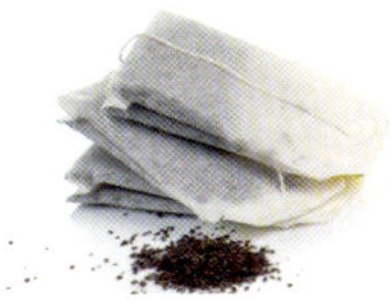

While the loose leaf teas described above are wonderful, most Americans drink tea packaged in bags bought at the supermarket. They enjoy the convenience and the fact that teabags infuse quickly. The reason for the quick infusion is that most bagged teas are comprised of fannings and dust. This sounds uninviting, but I can assure you that the manufacturers don't scoop the leftovers from the factory floor. These terms refer to the smallest leaves and tiniest broken pieces that remain at the end of the manufacturing process. Many of these little leaves taste very good. There is no shame in showing a preference for bagged tea, especially if you enjoy a strong flavor.

STORING TEA

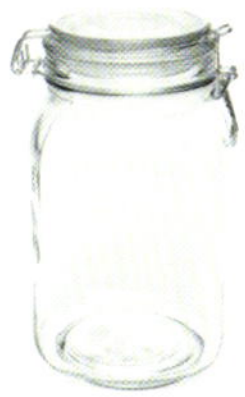

No matter what kind of tea you purchase, whether you buy it bagged or loose, you'll want to store it in an airtight container to preserve freshness. Black tea keeps longest–around a year. Oolong, green, and white teas have a shorter lifespan, anywhere from three-to-six months. If black tea goes stale, spread a thin layer on a sheet of paper for a few hours in a well-aired room. Unfortunately, the other types will degrade quickly if they undergo this treatment.

Serves 2

OCHAZUKE SOUP

If, after experimenting with the above suggestions, you still feel doubtful about the taste of green tea–although I can't imagine how anyone would–you can drink green tea as a soup. It fits as a potion, too, because it is liquid–that is, if you don't count the rice, fish, and vegetables. The qualities ascribed to this soup are very much in line with the reasons why we drink chicken soup and similar potions. In our respective cultures these soups represent the comforts of home. We drink them anytime, but especially when we aren't feeling well or after a night of revelry. Ochazuke soup is an easy recipe to prepare, too. You can vary it according to taste, or simply pop in juicy refrigerator leftovers. The word ochazuke means "tea pickle," so you can even add pickled vegetables if you wish. Here is a recipe.

Ingredients

1 cup cooked rice (If it's leftover rice, warm it in the microwave for a minute or so.)

4 ounces grilled salmon, cut into bite-size pieces (You can substitute cod or whitefish.)

1 cup hot green, brewed tea (Gyokuro makes an excellent choice, but any green tea will do.)

Directions

Place the warm rice in a bowl and mix in the salmon. Pour the green tea with some of its leaves over the mixture. Drink, and feel comforted and revived!

For extra flavor and variety: add ¼ cup of a pickled item like plums, ginger, carrots, and/or diced scallions. You can also sprinkle in shredded nori seaweed, salted salmon bits, bonito flakes, sesame seeds, crumbled rice crackers, soy sauce and/or wasabi.

Tea Potions and Your Health

Lu Yu, a Chinese monk widely proclaimed as "the saint of tea," wrote the first book (780 CE) to extol the medicinal virtues of this bewitching brew. In it, he declared that tea provides "vigor of body, contentment of mind, and determination of purpose," and that drinking tea cures ills as far-ranging as headache, depression, constipation, and sore muscles.

Today's promoters of tea—especially green tea—make pretty much the same claims. The popular press sometimes latches on to such reports and inflates the results for the consumption of readers eager to embrace a miracle cure. Since this is a book about potions and better health is one reason people drink them, in this part of the chapter I'll address some of the health claims made about tea.

Why Tea Makes a Healthy Potion

All tea contains more or less the same healthful substances. The differences in the way the various types are processed, coupled with where and how they are cultivated, makes for the variations. In general, green tea contains more concentrated healthy ingredients than black tea. Following is a list with short descriptions:

ANTIOXIDANTS

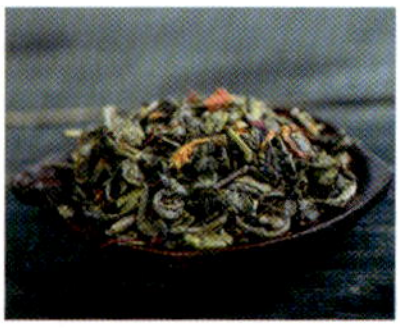

These substances help remove potentially damaging oxidizing agents in the blood. A class of antioxidants present in tea are called polyphenols. Polyphenols protect heart and blood vessels and reduce swelling and inflammation. The tannins in tea (described below) are also antioxidant. The antioxidants in 2 cups of black tea equal those contained in 1 glass of red wine, 7 of orange juice, or 20 cups of apple juice.

CATECHINS

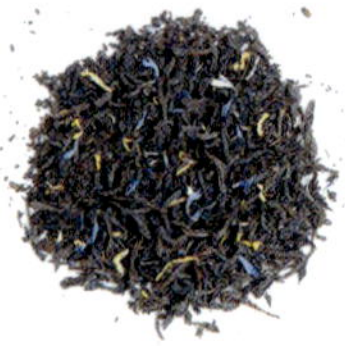

This class of antioxidants present in tea protects against human papilloma virus, cancers of the skin, esophagus, lungs, pancreas, prostate, cervix, and ovaries, and lowers the risk of heart attack.

EGCG

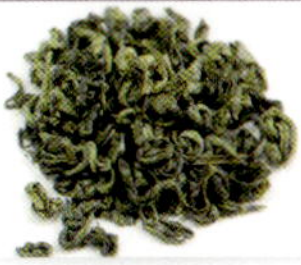

Otherwise known by the impressive name epigallocatechin-3-gallate, this flavonoid (a kind of antioxidant) found in green tea can keep free radicals from damaging and destroying cells and boost the immune system. It also helps strengthen bones and staves off osteoporosis.

FLUORIDE AND CHLOROPHYLL

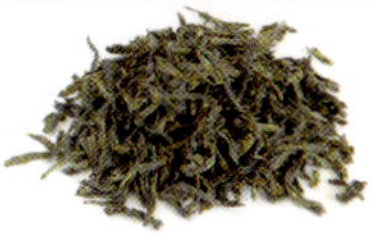

Green tea is rich in these substances, which are good for strengthening teeth and bones and stopping cavities and gum disease in their tracks.

CAFFEINE

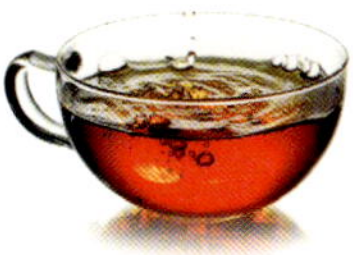

The caffeine content of tea, especially black tea, stimulates the nervous system, heart, and muscles by releasing certain chemicals into the brain that increase energy and improve cognitive functions. Oolong tea is especially good for helping to control various neurological diseases. Black tea contains theophylline, which speeds up heart rate and makes a person feel more alert.

VITAMINS AND MINERALS

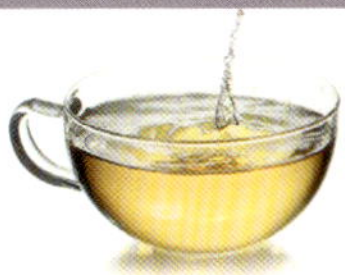

Tea contains many vitamins and minerals including A, B complex, C, D, K, and traces of manganese and amino acids.

Tea Is Not a Panacea

Tea is not a cure-all for every ailment. For example, there simply is not enough evidence to substantiate claims made for green tea's abilities to help with weight loss, lower high blood pressure, and prevent cancers of the colon and breast.

Doctors warn not to drink tea if you have, or are susceptible to, the following: anemia (or if you are vegetarian or vegan because the tannins in tea can interfere with iron absorption), already suffer from diabetes (although tea is also a diabetes preventative), glaucoma (tea increases the pressure inside the eye), irregular heartbeat, or high blood pressure. Since tea is a diuretic, drinking too much can flush from the system vitamins and minerals like calcium.

Tea also interferes with certain medications such as blood thinners. This is especially true for green tea. You should not drink black tea if you take stimulants like cocaine, amphetamines, ephedrine, nicotine, or any other drug that interacts with caffeine.

The tannins in tea that you may have heard about are not necessarily bad for you. In the first place, tea's tannins have nothing to do with tannic acid, which is used to tan leather. The tannins in tea are a wide class of polyphenols that lend the dark color, astringent flavor, body, and strength to black tea. They are the same tannins that are in red wine and have similar effects. Tannins can strengthen the immune system because they are antioxidant and antimicrobial. They can also help lower blood pressure and increase blood clotting.

Ingesting caffeine, which is especially present in black tea, while good in some respects, can cause nervousness, tremors, irregular heartbeat, vomiting, diarrhea, sleep disorders, ringing in the ears, heartburn, dizziness, anxiety, and increase bleeding risk. Caffeine consumption can worsen hormonal conditions that result in endometriosis, uterine fibroids, and cancers of breast, ovary, and uterus.

In tea's favor, the caffeine content of brewed tea is pretty much a lightweight compared to coffee. Here is the short list of caffeine amounts for brewed tea. The statistics come from the USDA National Nutrient Database for Standard Reference. (See Chapter 5 for information on coffee's caffeine content.)

Tea Type	Brewed Ounces	Average Caffeine Content
White Tea	8 ounces	15 mg
Green Tea	8 ounces	20 mg
Oolong Tea	8 ounces	30 mg
Black Tea	8 ounces	48 mg

Although the caffeine in tea activates the respiratory and central nervous systems as well as the kidneys, tea also contains the mild muscle relaxants theophylline and theobromine. It seems you can relax but remain alert when you drink tea. Rather like having your cake and eating it, too! How the caffeine in tea affects you largely depends on your health and daily tea intake.

Here is an easy way to reduce the amount of caffeine you ingest in tea by one-half. It is a known fact that caffeine dissolves in boiling water. After brewing the tea, let it steep for a couple of minutes, and then discard the cup's contents. If you don't want to throw away the tea you can fertilize your camellias and rhododendrons with the water. Brew a second cup using the same bag or leaves. Steep, and *voilà!* Your cup of tea will now contain approximately fifty percent less caffeine.

Tea Trends

Beyond the Green

While tea is as old as the Himalayas, many Americans have only recently discovered the joys of taking tea. And as things usually go in our consumer-oriented society, this interest has led to several new products, as well as traditional products repackaged and marketed for contemporary times. Here's the scoop on some popular trends.

Gourmet Teas

In this category are various specialty teas sought after by connoisseurs. For example, Artisan Teas are premium, whole leaf teas of any of the four types. They are processed in small batches and hand-sewn into rosettes. A gourmet might choose one of these teas to celebrate a special occasion or individual. The rosette is placed in the bottom of the cup, boiling water is poured over it, and the bud slowly opens to reveal an anemone or peony flower in full bloom.

Another specialty, Functional Tea, borrows its name from sports medicine. These teas are meant to appeal to health-conscious gourmets. The manufacturers add vitamins, minerals, amino acids, and other substances purported to keep a person healthy and enhance athletic performance. The teas are packaged conveniently, often in single servings, and sold in much the same way as sports drinks.

Yet another type of tea fancied by connoisseurs is Puerh (also spelled "pu-erh" and "puer"). This tea is harvested from ancient trees in the southern mountains of Yunnan Province, China. For three months or more the moist, whole leaves undergo microbial fermentation underground. The process makes the fermenting tea resemble a rotting compost heap. Never fear: fermentation is constantly monitored for temperature and moisture. The result is a dark brown-colored brewed tea with an earthy flavor. Puerh tea is celebrated as the ultimate digestive aid.

Tea Cocktails and Liqueurs

Some may take their tea in the form of a cocktail or liqueur. These drinks are marketed to appeal to a hip, young generation who want to relax after work with an alcoholic beverage and ingest some vitamins and antioxidants in the bargain. A true tea connoisseur would probably blanch at the prospect of adding alcohol to tea, citing how it destroys tea's delicate aroma and taste. Nonetheless, these beverages have made a big splash in the US and Europe. The tradition goes back to at least the nineteenth century when, in Great Britain, people combined hot tea with rum or whiskey, honey, and spices. Family and friends cozied around the fire on blustery nights, cold hands clutched around their cups, sipping the brew they called "hot toddy."

Tea as Food

Another chic trend is to treat tea as food. Again, this tradition harkens back 3,000 years to the early days of tea consumption in Asia. For example, tea leaves can be steamed or stir-fried with sesame oil and eaten like spinach. In this way, the diner salvages the fiber, carotene, vitamin E, protein, and much of the chlorophyll in the leaves. Sauces and marinades can also be concocted from the leaves. Asians even smoke food in the leaves. Other products with tea or tealeaf ingredients include broth, bread, cake, candy, and gum.

Bubble Tea for the Youth Market

Here's a unique way to introduce children to the joys of taking tea (although adults can enjoy it, too). Bubble tea was invented in Taiwan in the 1980s by a street vendor who wanted to draw children and others to his cart. He set up outside schools and businesses on hot afternoons when the workday was ending. He flavored cold tea with sweet fruit, added milk and ice, and created a shake that bubbled to the top of the glass. Around the same time, another Taiwanese vendor decided to add chewy, white, black, or clear-colored tapioca pearls to the concoction to make the shake even more visually appealing. Bubble Tea is poured in a clear glass so the marble-size pearls can be admired. The tea drinker sucks up the pearls through a special fat straw. This very sweet tea is sometimes called Pearl Tea or Boba Tea.

Sweet Tea Southern Style

Speaking of sweet Bubble Tea reminds me of an experience a couple of years ago on a cruise along the Danube River. After returning to the boat from a long day of exploration, the crew had plenty of iced water, carbonated beverages, and cold tea for us to drink. I filled my glass rapidly and took a long, greedy gulp, and . . . almost gagged. The tea had been pre-sweetened! This was my startling introduction to Sweet Tea.

Sweet Tea is not exactly a new trend since it has been drunk throughout the South since the nineteenth century. If my experience on the Danube and all the sweet ready-to-drink teas (another trend) stacked on grocery store shelves are any indication, this way of taking tea has spread throughout the country. According to blogs I've read, many Canadians, despite the cold climate, also drink Sweet Iced Tea with their meals. Sweet Tea is made from iced green or black tea. The sweetener is added during the brewing process. For me, the sugariness obliterates the natural aroma and flavor, but millions of Southerners will undoubtedly disagree.

Chai Tea

Chai is my very favorite kind of tea. My husband, who breakfasts at a nearby café, brings me home a cup of it every morning. Also called Masala Chai, this fragrant blend of black or green tea brewed with milk, sugar, and spices hails from India, where it is a venerable tradition. A few decades ago, you rarely found it served anywhere in the West, but since it was "discovered," demand has soared. Now you can find Chai as a dry blend, in teabag form or even ready-to-drink at the grocery, and it is served at most coffeehouses. On a recent trip to Oxford, England, I was elated to see Chai offered at the coach stop. In my opinion, a Chai potion makes one of the healthiest and most pleasant ways to start the day. If you brew yours from green tea, you'll reap green tea's health benefits along with the calcium and vitamin D found in milk. Then there are the spices. Besides tasting good, cardamom, cinnamon, cloves, coriander, cumin, ginger, nutmeg and pepper–some or all of which are included in the mix–are good for you. (For more information on these spices, see Chapter 6.)

Serves 1

Brand New Day CHAI

Photograph by C. Nathan Pulley Photography

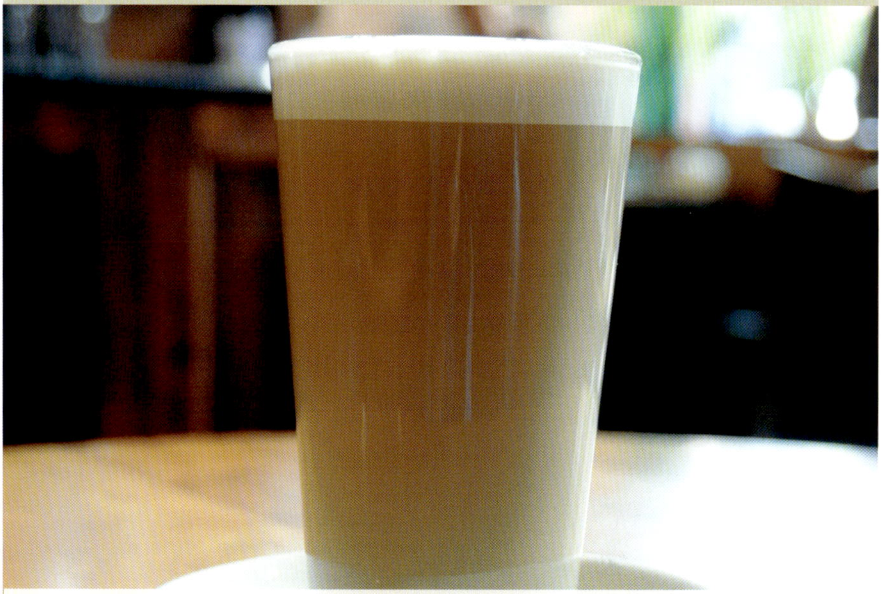

Here's a simple recipe for whipping up your own chai. Drink it in the morning and the spices will energize you for the day ahead. Drink it at night and the milk and vanilla will lull you to sleep. *Photographed at the Trident bookstore and Café.*

Ingredients

1 cup Chai, brewed from a Chai teabag in milk

¼ teaspoon vanilla granules (if you can't find them, use vanilla extract)

¼ teaspoon fresh ginger, grated

¼ teaspoon cinnamon, ground

¼ teaspoon green or black cardamom pod, crushed

⅛ teaspoon Irish moss (Irish moss is loaded with nutrients and adds texture to the drink.)

Dash of clove powder

1 cinnamon stick

Directions

Blend all ingredients, stir with a cinnamon stick, and drink.

To save time I like to make up a small spice jarful of the dry ingredients in advance and add 1 teaspoonful each time to the brew.

Iced Tea

In spite of the popularity of the foregoing trends, a majority of Americans drink their tea iced. Eighty-five percent of the tea we consume is iced black tea, and we gulp it down year round. Exactly who and when iced tea was invented is hotly disputed, but the custom seems to have taken hold during the nineteenth century in both the US and in Britain as a non-alcoholic alternative to green tea punches.

Whether you brew iced tea from loose leaves or bags, be sure to make it twice as strong as your beverage tea. The ice you add will dilute the brew by half. If you wish, add sugar while the brew is hot so it readily dissolves.

Makes 1 Quart

Fast Microwave ICED TEA

The following recipe for preparing iced tea is especially handy when guests drop by and you need to give them iced tea right away. It uses bags and a microwave oven. Remember to remove the staples so they don't arc or create sparks in the oven.

Ingredients

- 4 cup hot water, split
- 4 teabags
- Sweetner to taste
- Ice
- 1 lemon, sliced (if desired)

Directions

Place 1 cup of hot water with 4 teabags in a microwave-safe container. Cook on high for 2 minutes. Remove the tea bags from the tea. Sweeten while hot, if desired. Next place 3 cups of cold water in a 1 quart pitcher and add the hot tea; stir well. Pour over ice to serve. Garnish with a slice of lemon, if desired.

Steeped in Tea: Brewing the Perfect Cuppa

As the Japanese tea ceremony attests, brewing and drinking tea can be an art in itself, and many benefits can be derived from performing this daily ritual. As many ways to brew tea exist as there are cultures in the world—perhaps more. Most experts agree that the best way to enjoy a good cup of tea is to prepare an infusion. This consists of the following steps:

1. Boil 1 cupful of water (although some gourmets advise to wait 2 minutes for the water to cool before adding the tea so not to scorch the leaves and end up with a flat-tasting brew).
2. Pour the boiling water over 1 teaspoonful of fresh leaves, ½ teaspoonful of dried, or 1 teabag and
3. Steep the brew in a nonmetal container for up to five minutes.

4. If you use a teabag, remove it. Never squeeze a teabag into the cup to extract the rest of the liquid, as it will taste yucky (a highly technical term!).
5. If you use loose leaves, pour the tea through a strainer into a fresh cup. Add sugar, honey, or molasses, and lemon or milk if desired.
6. Stir once, and drink immediately. Natural soft, filtered water makes a superior cup of tea.

Teapot Tea

Many amusing old wives' tales have evolved around teapot brewing. One superstition warns not to stir the pot counter clockwise or you will incite trouble. Another claims that if you spill some tea while pouring you will be lucky.

Superstition aside, brewing a fine pot of tea is truly an art form, but one you can master easily once you learn a few basics.

1. Start by warming the teapot. Pour hot water into it, swish it around and then pour it out.
2. Next comes the tea. Edward Bramah, tea broker, entrepreneur, true tea connoisseur, and founder of the Bramah Museum of Tea and Coffee in London, wrote numerous articles on tea over his lifetime. Bramah insisted that the tea should always be a good quality loose leaf, not a teabag. He recommended Broken Orange Pekoe (BOP) or a second-flush (second harvest) Indian Assam as pleasing to most people. Put in 1 teaspoonful of leaves for each person you are serving and an extra one for the pot.
3. Fill the pot with 1 cup per guest of fresh, filtered hot water.
4. Stir the leaves and let them steep for up to five minutes.
5. Place the sugar and milk or lemon slice in each guest's cup if they wish it, and pour the tea through a mesh strainer.
6. Once the pot is empty, refill it with more hot water so the leaves continue to release strength and flavor. Cover the pot with a cozy (an insulated cotton cover) to keep the tea piping hot. Always discard cold tea left in a cup before refilling it.

If you prefer teabags, place one in the pot for each guest you plan to serve. Proceed as with loose tea, only remove the bags after you have poured. If you leave teabags in the hot water too long the tea will taste astringent. You can follow this procedure with a single cup as well. I like to cover my cup with a saucer while it steeps so the essential oils don't dissipate.

Tea Color Potions

Chapter 1 introduced the subject of how color relates to potion-crafting by exerting psychological and physical effects on the human body. I have also alluded to tea potions and color throughout this chapter. There are four basic tea colors: clear-to-whitish or yellow, green, reddish-brown, and brownish-orange.

The color of the tea and the way it is processed combine to create specific effects on the body:

WHITE

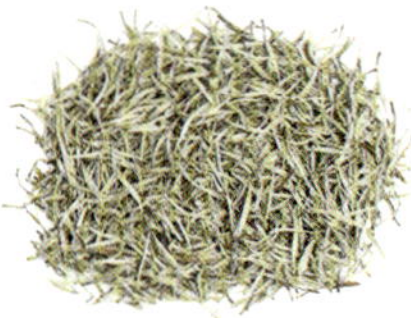

White teas are relaxing and can be drunk to soothe frazzled nerves and put you in a receptive frame of mind for meditation.

GREEN

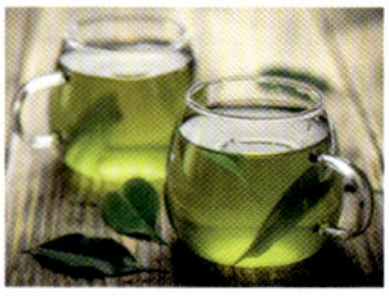

Green represents harmony of body, mind, and spirit. Green teas are often drunk to achieve better health.

BLACK

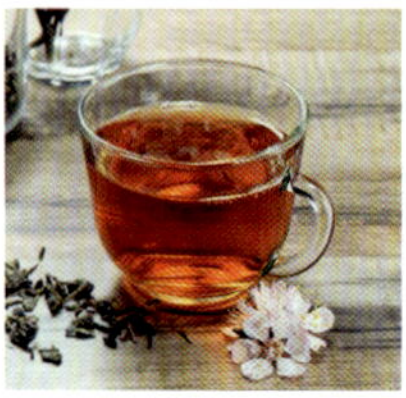

Black teas, which when brewed often turn red or orange in color, can be drunk to receive an infusion of energy and alertness. They also contain the most caffeine.

BROWN

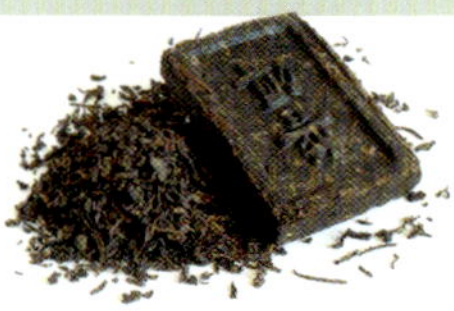

Teas that brew *brown* in the cup can aid focus on goals and improve digestion. Following are tea recipes that rely on color to help produce certain results.

Serves 2

Valentine's Day WHITE PEONY TEA

You can whip up this simple recipe in no time. Share it with your special someone in front of a cozy fire. It both relaxes and sparks passion due to some colorful ingredients:

Ingredients

- 2 cups boiling water
- 1 teaspoon loose White Peony or any white tea
- ½ teaspoon red rose buds
- ½ teaspoon candied passion fruit pieces, cut up fairly small. (If you have trouble finding passion fruit pieces, substitute dried, diced apricots.)
- Water, boiling

Directions

Place equal portions of the mixture of the three items at the bottom of 2 teacups. Pour boiling water over the tea and steep for 2 minutes. Stir well and let the solid matter settle on the bottom. Do not remove the leaves before drinking; most will stay at the bottom.

Serves 2

Rise 'n' Shine TEA

This combination of stimulating ingredients and bright orange color will fire both mind and body for the day ahead. It renders 2 cups, in case you want a second pick-me-up later.

Ingredients

- 2 cups hot water
- 1 teaspoon Orange Pekoe tea
- ¼ teaspoon nettles
- ¼ teaspoon instant ginseng tea
- ¼ teaspoon guaraná seeds, crushed

Directions

Brew all ingredients for 3 minutes and strain away the herbs before drinking.

Serves about 4

Chase Away the Blues
TEA SMOOTHIE

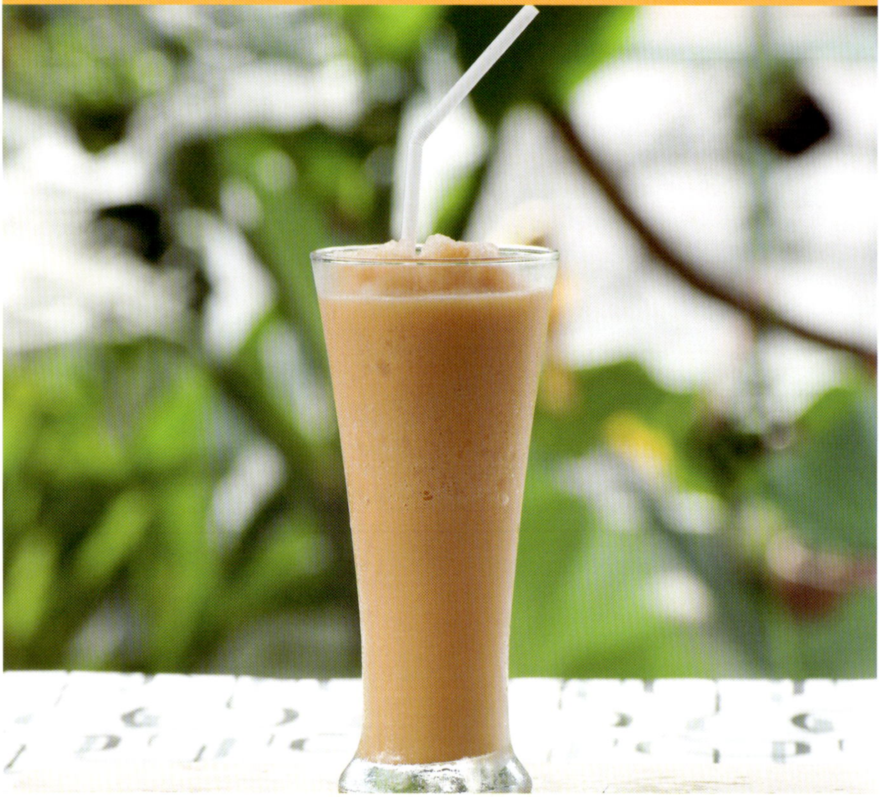

This smoothie looks and tastes like a Creamsicle, and is guaranteed to lift your spirits.

Ingredients

- 1 6-ounce can orange juice, frozen concentrate
- 1 cup brewed green tea, cooled
- 1 cup whole milk
- 1 teaspoon vanilla extract
- ½ teaspoon almond extract
- 6 ice cubes

Directions

Place all of the ingredients into a blender, cover, and blend until smooth. Serve at once.

Now that we've covered my personal favorite beverage potion, it's time to turn to most Americans' favorite potion–you guessed it–coffee.

Chapter 5

SO YOU'RE A COFFEE DRINKER, EH?

Making Sense of the Grounds

If you enjoy coffee as much as T. S. Eliot, this chapter is for you. Here you will find ways to incorporate this rich, aromatic brew into your ever-expanding armory of potions. The chapter provides information on coffee, including an overview of coffee history, its nutritional value, bean varieties, coffee drinks, recipes, and anecdotes to share with other coffee lovers. At the end, I present an unusual and entertaining way to enjoy your coffee by showing how to divine your future in the grounds.

I have measured out my life with coffee spoons.
–T. S. Eliot (1888–1965), English author of "The Love Song of J. Alfred Prufrock"

Background on the Grounds

Coffee is produced from the red berries of a small jungle tree which, like tea, is grown as a bush under cultivation. The grayish-green or yellow beans are grouped in twos inside the berry. When ripe, they are harvested, fermented, washed, dried, roasted, and finally ground. Peaberry coffee is made from the small percentage of single, round beans found in the pods; hence the name.

Sources agree that the coffee tree hails from Africa, probably current-day Ethiopia. As with tea, lively legends have developed around coffee's origin. In one story, a Dervish who crossed a king was left to die in a cave in the barren terrain outside of Mocha, Yemen. A bird singing on a coffee tree branch drew the victim's attention to the bush's red berries. Thinking he had nothing to lose, the man ate the berries, which he found amazingly flavorful. He gained sustenance and strength and survived to extol the energizing virtues of the coffee plant.

Another story claims that Ethiopian shepherds discovered the bean's revitalizing properties when they observed how joyfully their flock scampered around after munching the fruit. It is said that King Solomon learned of coffee's healing powers from no less a figure than the Archangel Gabriel, the healing aspect of God.

Coffee was unknown to the ancient cultures of Egypt, Greece, and Rome. By around 575–850 CE this tree of the Madder family was cultivated in the Red Sea region. Arab traders introduced coffee to the Mediterranean countries in the West.

Imbibing the brew and interpreting the grounds soon caught on as a captivating form of in-home entertainment. The beverage became so beloved that Muslim clerics of the era, who had already managed to ban alcohol, failed abysmally in their efforts to prohibit coffee consumption. Ever since, coffee drinking has become an ingrained part of the social fabric in Muslim culture.

Pope Sanctifies Coffee

As coffee's fame spread to Europe, the Roman Catholic Church cast a jaundiced eye on the infidels' black potion. One fine day, Pope Clement VII decided to sample the foul liquid to see what kind of devil he was up against. After taking the first sip, he proclaimed that since Satan had gone to the trouble to concoct such a delicious drink, it would be a shame to leave it for the heathens. The solution? He baptized coffee and sanctified it as a "proper Christian drink."

Coffee Cultivation Goes Worldwide

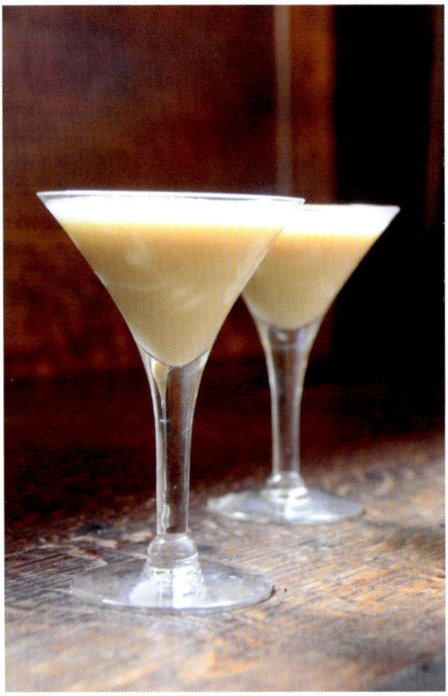

Photograph by C. Nathan Pulley Photography

Irish Coffee Cream Cordial.

Although the Arabs struggled to keep the secrets of coffee cultivation and preparation under wraps, eventually a French naval officer smuggled a plant to Martinique, where he sequestered the rare and valuable botanical under armed guard. Alas, the Frenchman was also doomed in his attempt to conceal the mysteries of coffee. Soon, coffee cultivation had spread throughout the Caribbean and into Brazil, where it became a principal export crop.

Today, coffee is grown around the world wherever the climate is favorable. Plantations thrive in such far-flung locations as Brazil, Jamaica, Martinique, Ethiopia, Kenya, Mexico, Hawaii, Sumatra, New Guinea, Uganda, Yemen, India, Tanzania, Zimbabwe, Central America, Vietnam, and Columbia.

After the Boston Tea Party and the American Revolution, coffee replaced tea in Yankee hearts, and it hasn't budged much since. Explorers, pioneers, and cowboys fueled themselves with coffee on their marches across the country to fulfill their Manifest Destiny. During Prohibition, coffee even substituted for liquor as a temperance drink.

Each day, 400 million cups of coffee are consumed. That's over nine pounds (4.2 kilograms) per capita each year! One-third of North American tap water for drinking is estimated to be expended in brewing coffee. Statistics from 2013 show that Starbucks uses 93 million gallons of milk every year to create its famous coffee drinks.

Varieties of Coffee

The two major species of coffee tree are the *Coffea arabica,* and *C. robusta*. Coffee made from the first species tastes rich and flavorful, but contains less caffeine. The *robusta* species renders a more acidic, highly caffeinated, bitter brew. Within these two species varieties are mostly categorized according to the location where they are grown.

As with tea, micro-variations in climate conditions, altitude, rainfall, and soil greatly impact the flavor of the beans and make for different varieties. For example, from Brazil hail the delicately flavored Bourbon Santos, Maragogipe giants, Mundo Novo, Cerrado, Caturra, Yellow Bourbon, Bahia, and the more acidic Rio beans. Indonesian Kopi Luwak is an exotic variety that costs as much as $600 per pound. It is only recommended for the most adventurous coffee aficionados as it is gathered from the excrement of the palm civet mongoose, whose diet is largely composed of coffee beans. The civet's gastric juices supposedly neutralize the acidity and bitterness, resulting in a smooth, sweet-tasting coffee. Or so I'm told.

Coffee Roasts

How coffee is roasted also impacts the flavor. For example, you can buy a Colombia Supremo Dark Roast, an Espresso Roast, a French Vienna, or even a Mocha-Java roast. If drinking too much coffee gives you heartburn, or if you are caffeine-sensitive, or pregnant and trying to cut back, go with the darker roasts. Besides having a better flavor, they contain less caffeine and acid.

Coffee enthusiasts may wish to purchase and roast their own beans. Although detailing the procedure for roasting green beans lies beyond the scope of this book–if you roast your own, you will pay approximately fifteen-to-twenty-five percent less for your cup of java. Be sure to store the beans in a dark, cool, dry place so they don't grow mold.

Coffee and Your Health

It is said that laughter is the best medicine. If coffee puts you in as good a humor as it did for Clark Gable, it must be very good medicine, indeed. Evidently Solomon and Gabriel, whom you read about in the history section, agreed, for they proclaimed coffee a formidable healer of body, mind, and spirit. Besides the well-known stimulating effects of caffeine, medical science has discovered other virtues for the coffee bean. Before I exalt coffee's merits, let's start with some caffeine facts.

Caffeine: Angel or Devil?

Ever wonder how much caffeine you swallow with your morning coffee? According to the USDA National Nutrient Database for Standard Reference, you will ingest 90–150 milligrams (mg) with each cup of drip-brewed coffee, 65–125 mg for percolated, and 60–80 mg if you prefer instant. All of these amounts far exceed those you learned about in Chapter 4 for various kinds of tea. Even decaffeinated coffee comes up with between 8.6–13.9 milligrams per cup.

How does the caffeine in coffee compare with other caffeine-infused items? Well, it turns out there's a lot of caffeine in coffee. Here's a comparison chart:

Item	Quantity	Average Caffeine Content
Coca-Cola™	12 ounces	34 mg
Starbucks™ coffee	Double shot 8 ounces	160 mg
Cold relief pill	1 tablet	30 mg
Rockstar™ energy drink	8 ounces	80 mg
Stay-awake pill	1 tablet	100 mg
Black tea 8 ounces	8 ounces	48 mg
White tea	8 ounces	15 mg

For some people coffee consumption causes irritability, nervousness, muscle tremors, nausea, headaches, restlessness, increased need to urinate (because it is a mild diuretic), and insomnia. Caffeine-sensitive folks probably learned long ago to stay away from coffee. Fortunately, these disagreeable symptoms do not affect everyone. Through chemical reactions that occur in the brain when a person drinks coffee, it is possible to build a tolerance to the caffeine so that the negative effects are not as impactful. A major study has even shown that among inveterate coffee drinkers, there are far fewer incidences of suicide than in total abstainers. Go figure!

I suppose how caffeine affects you largely hinges on your individual body chemistry and how much you drink. If you suffer from cystic fibrosis, high blood pressure, osteoporosis, or heart arrhythmia, caffeine may aggravate your symptoms. Certain medications and herbal supplements also interact negatively with caffeine. If you drink coffee and also take Theophylline, a drug that relaxes bronchial airways, you may experience heart palpitations, nausea, or vomiting. Some antibacterial medications like Ciprofloxacin and Noroxin can increase the length of time the effects of the caffeine stay in your body. Even the herbal supplement Echinacea, taken to prevent colds, may increase the damaging effects of caffeine in your body. Finally, scores of epidemiological studies have shown that high caffeine consumption in pregnant women contributes to lower birth weights and increased incidences of birth defects in newborns. How much coffee do the experts consider safe to drink? Two to four cups of brewed coffee per day is not considered harmful, and even has health benefits.

Coffee and Nutrition

If experts agree that limited coffee consumption is the way to go, why include this beverage in a wholesome potions book? Besides its popularity and the taste factor, coffee has a lot going for it in the health department. As the anonymous coffee lover quoted above cogently surmises, the caffeine in coffee alleviates fatigue, increases alertness, and improves concentration and focus by stimulating the central nervous system. Because it increases respiration and the action of the heart, coffee makes a valuable tool to fight overdoses from alcohol, morphine, marijuana, and barbiturates. Caffeine also enhances athletic performance. Coffee is a stimulant for adults, but mixed with warm milk, the beverage has been prescribed by doctors to calm children, especially those afflicted with ADD. As with any home remedy, I advise you to consult a doctor before trying this therapy.

Both coffee and tea are advertised as anti-cancer beverages. Specifically, coffee's caffeine content sloughs off cancerous skin cells and protects against colon and liver cancer as well as Type 2 diabetes. The effects of Parkinson's and Alzheimer's diseases are ameliorated by coffee consumption and the caffeine helps prevent gallstones from forming as well. Caffeine may help manage asthma, although more studies need to be done in this area.

The above-quoted anonymous coffee drinker's tongue-in-cheek plug for coffee as a vitamin is not too far off the mark. Coffee contains the minerals magnesium and chromium, which help the body use insulin; hence the link to diabetes control. It also contains antioxidants. As yet scientists have not determined whether those plucky free-radical fighters actually make it into the bloodstream.

Now that you're undoubtedly convinced of the magical restorative qualities of this beverage, let's move on to the fun part–coffee drinks and recipes.

Coffee Drinks

Even though I'm a confirmed tea drinker, I confess a fascination with the luscious-looking coffee concoctions that parade by in the cafés. I've been so enchanted by these fluffy, creamy delights that more than once I've yearned to sample a few. Trouble is, when I queue up, I'm flummoxed by the plethora of the different creations on offer and don't know what to request. If you have found yourself in the same hot water, here are a few definitions to help you select a drink that strikes your fancy. The list is not exhaustive, but does include the most common drinks you'll find at your local café.

AMERICANO

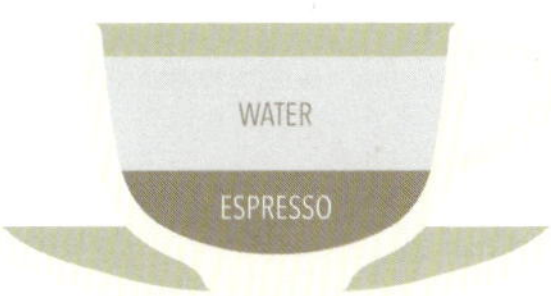

A single shot of espresso mixed with seven ounces of hot water. The name in Italian is a dig against North Americans, who at one time were considered incapable of drinking an entire espresso without watering it down. North Americans, take heart! We're not the only culture to be maligned as pitiable coffee drinkers. Dame Agatha Christie, the famous mystery writer, was an Englishwoman who traveled widely in the Middle East and Africa. She once quipped that, "Coffee in England always tastes like a chemistry experiment."

AU LAIT

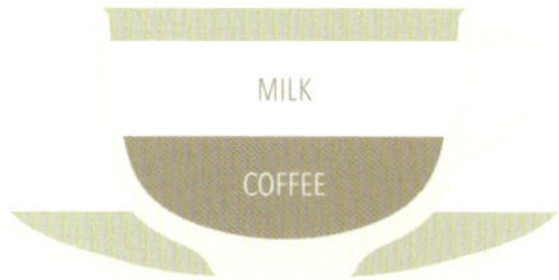

Café au lait is prepared from equal parts regular brewed coffee and warm, creamy milk. Some foam may be left on top, and many *au lait* drinkers add sweetener.

BLACK COFFEE

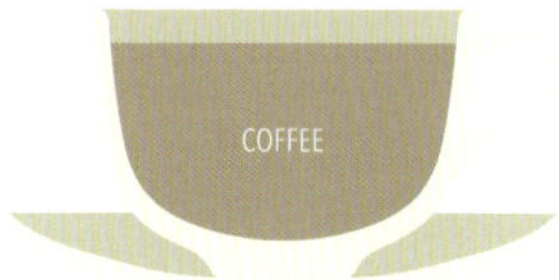

As the name implies, this coffee is served straight without milk. It can be drip brewed, French pressed, or percolated. Its opposite number is White Coffee, which is brewed as above with the addition of milk.

BREVA

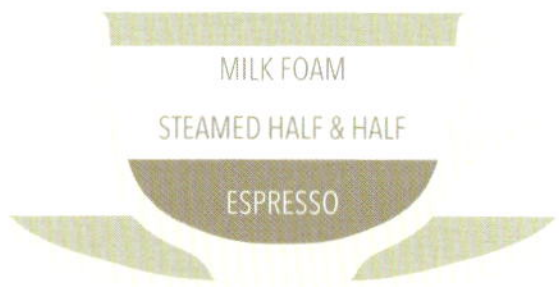

Here we're talking about a cappuccino made with half-and-half milk that gives the brew a creamier flavor.

CAPPUCCINO

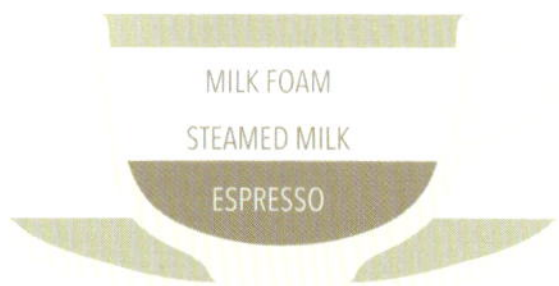

An espresso mixed with hot frothed milk or cream, and often flavored with cinnamon. The Italian word originates in the likeness of this drink to the color of a Capuchin monk's habit.

ESPRESSO

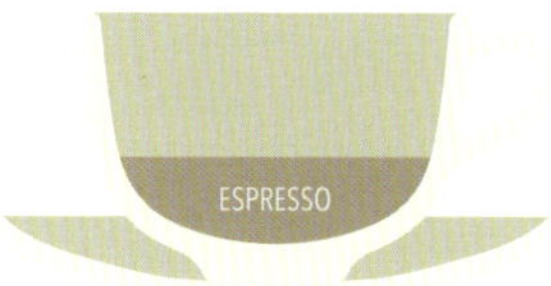

Probably the most common coffee drink you'll find at a café. It consists of coffee brewed by forcing hot water or steam through finely ground, dark roasted coffee beans. A single shot of espresso is used to make most coffee drinks. The term is based on the assumption that the coffee is made to order on the spot at the customer's request.

ESPRESSO CON PANNA

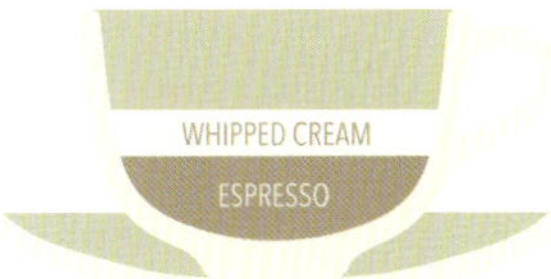

As the Italian name implies, a single shot of espresso topped with whipped cream.

FLAVORED COFFEES

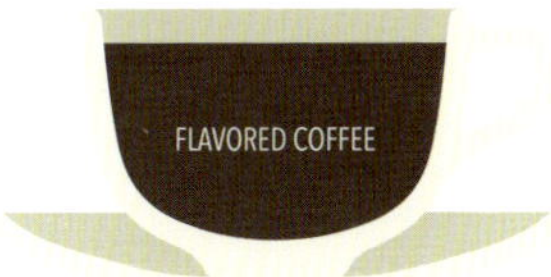

From time to time, some drinkers like to add extracts, syrups, and/or spices to their coffee to impart a bit of sparkle. The most popular addition is chocolate in the form of syrup or grated over the top of the drink. Other favorites include Italian syrups, cinnamon, and nutmeg.

FRAPPE

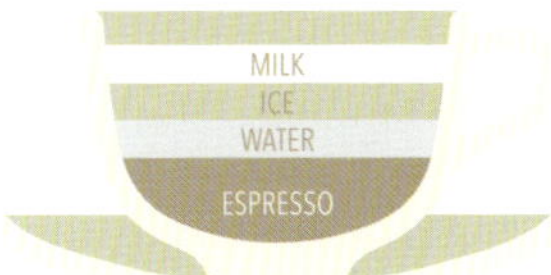

A summery drink resembling a smoothie. It is made from either cold espresso or 1 to 2 teaspoons of instant coffee. Add water, ice, sugar, and milk, and blend. Pour the mixture into a tall glass and enjoy.

ICED COFFEE

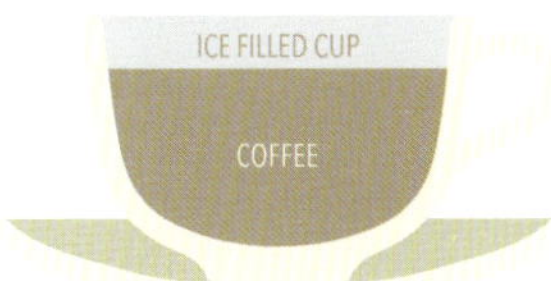

This drink reflects Americans' obsession with cold beverages. It is an Americano with ice, and sometimes milk and sugar, according to taste. Here's a recipe.

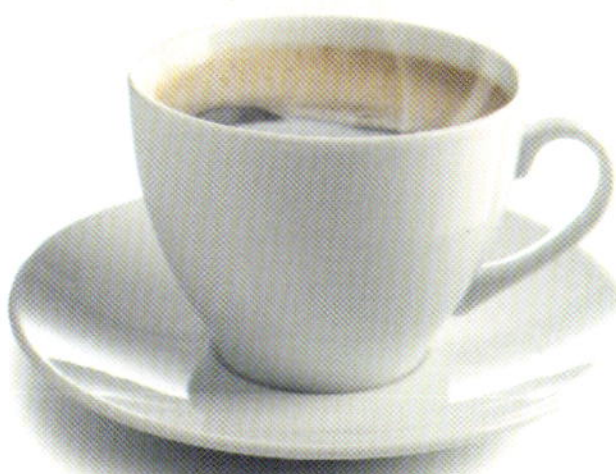

ICED COFFEE

Serves 1

Ingredients

- 1 cup chilled coffee, brewed extra strong (since you're going to use ice to dilute it)
- 1 tablespoon caramel syrup (Personally, I think everything tastes better with caramel.)
- ½ cup milk
- Demerara sugar to taste
- ½ teaspoon vanilla extract
- 1 cup ice
- Whipped cream (optional topping)

Directions

Mix all of the ingredients in a blender until smooth. Pour into a tall glass. If you top it with whipped cream, drizzle more caramel syrup over it. Now sit back on your deck and slurp away!

INSTANT COFFEE

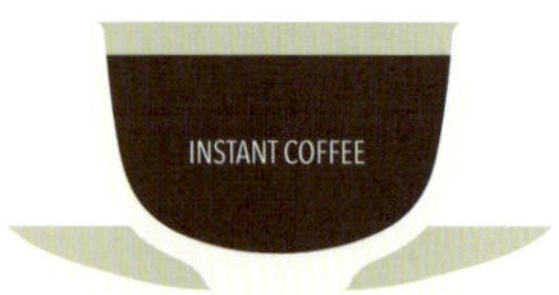

The grounds are freeze-dried to transform them into soluble powder or granules. Although the resulting quality of the coffee is not as rich-tasting as brewed, instant coffee is convenient for preparing smoothies and other potions.

IRISH COFFEE

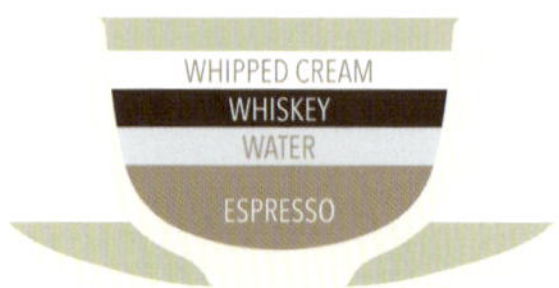

Irish coffee is a favorite after-dinner drink served in a goblet, cup, or mug of coffee drip brewed, percolated, or French pressed. Add a couple tablespoons of Irish whiskey and top it with whipped cream, my mother used to put 2 teaspoons of turbinado sugar (described in Chapter 6) in the bottom of each goblet, add the whiskey, and stir in just enough hot coffee to dissolve the sugar before filling up the goblet with more coffee.

LATTE

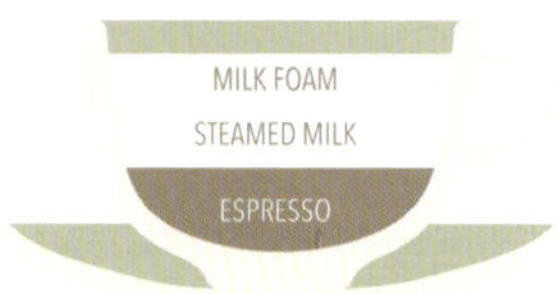

Caffè Latte is usually made from one-third espresso and ⅔ hot, steamed milk. Some like to add more than one shot of espresso, and it is often drunk without sugar. Usually no foam is left on top.

LUNGO

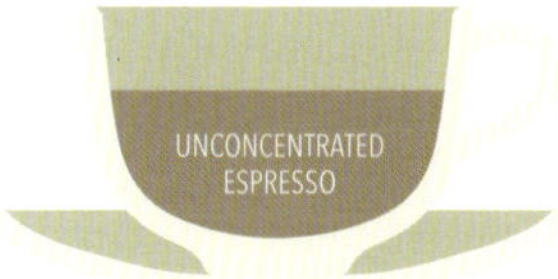

A barista prepares a Lungo by pressing twice as much water as usual through the coffee grounds for one shot of espresso. The result is a 2-to-3-ounce shot.

MACCHIATO

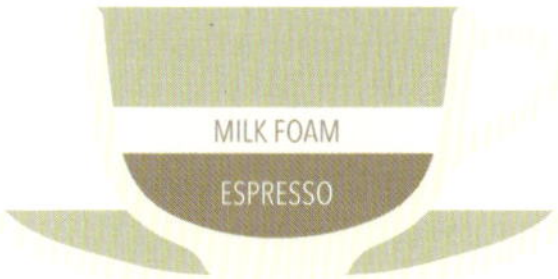

The definition of a true macchiato is hotly disputed. In Italian the word means "marked with spots." One description of the drink calls for a single shot of espresso with a dash (some say a small dollop) of hot or cold steamed milk dotted on top. Another source claims that you should dot 1-2 teaspoons of steamed milk over the top. Variations of this drink include one that adds caramel.

MOCHA

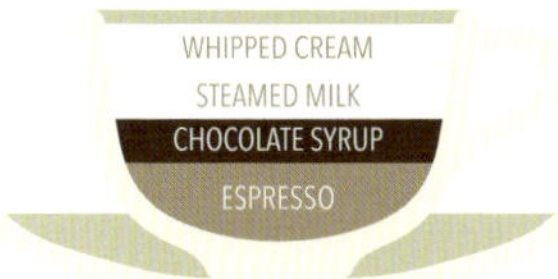

A cappuccino or latte with the addition of chocolate syrup. The syrup makes the coffee flavor less intense and sweeter. This is why mocha is often referred to as a coffee "starter" drink for the uninitiated.

RISTRETTO

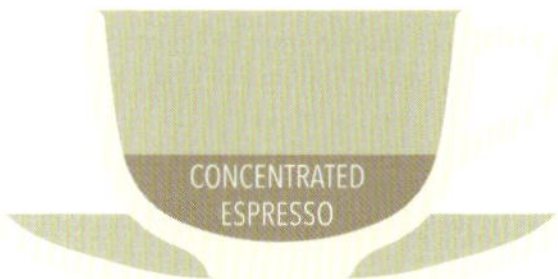

With a lungo, more water is pulled through the grounds, but with a ristretto, less water is pushed through, even though the barista takes the same amount of time to make the pull. This process renders a 0.75 ounce shot.

TURKISH COFFEE *(also called Greek Coffee)*

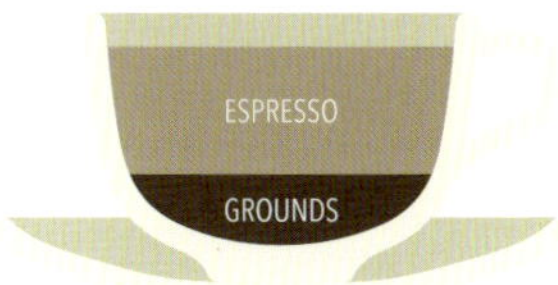

The kind preferred for coffee ground reading (described below). It leaves a thick, muddy trail of grounds in the bottom of the cup that makes easily interpretable images. Often Turkish coffee is drunk with the addition of sugar and spices such as cinnamon and cardamom.

Photograph by C. Nathan Pulley Photography

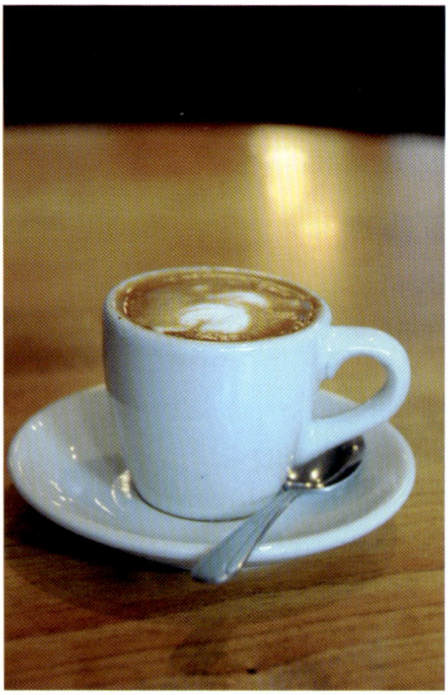

Macchiato. Photo shot at The Trident Bookstore and Café.

No matter what form of coffee gives you pleasure, most experts agree that it should be served at 155°-170° F degrees. Any hotter, and you risk evaporating the essential oils, which give coffee its distinctive flavor and aroma. If you take milk or cream in your coffee, but don't like the cooling effects, preheat it before adding to the cup.

Coffee Potions

Under nutritional benefits of coffee, I discussed how this drink can keep you alert and focused. Following is a coffee smoothie potion to help sharpen your wits. This recipe also takes advantage of additional ingredients claimed to hone intellectual skills.

Serves 2

COFFEE SMOOTHIE

Ingredients

- 1 cup coffee, strongly brewed and cooled
- 1 cup cold milk
- ½ frozen banana, chopped (for increased energy)
- ½ teaspoon vanilla extract (for mental clarity)
- ¼ teaspoon almond extract (for wisdom)
- ¼ teaspoon coconut extract (for strength)
- Sugar to taste. *
- 2 cups ice cubes
- Cinnamon, sprinkle

Directions

Blend all ingredients well. Add ice little by little, blending each time until you achieve the frothy smoothness you desire. Pour into tall glasses and sprinkle with cinnamon, a spice which is claimed to increase knowledge, aid memory, fire inspiration, and promote self-development.

* Because the banana is sweet, you may not want to add sugar. If you do, I recommend using demerara sugar for this recipe.

Serves 2

MOCHA YOGURT SMOOTHIE

Photograph by C. Nathan Pulley Photography

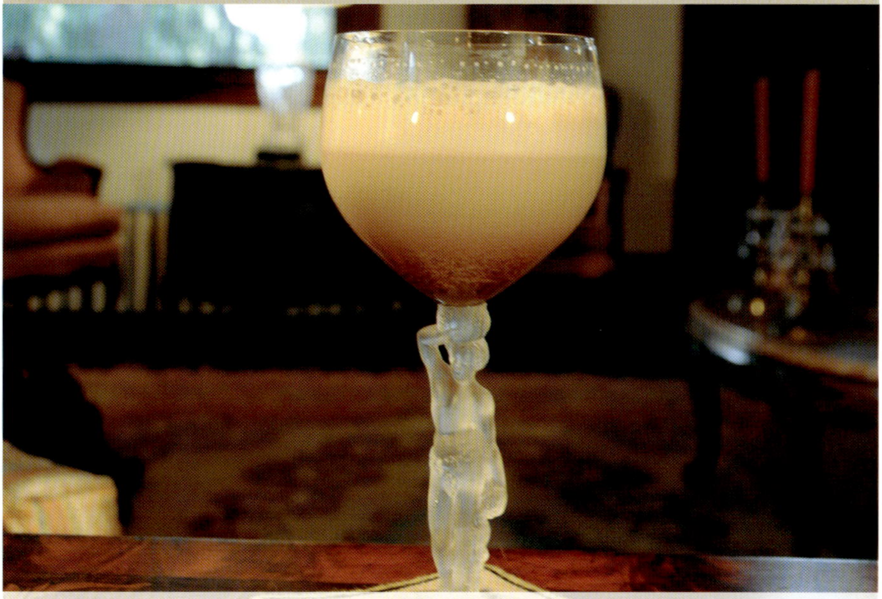

This recipe combines your favorite coffee with sinfully delicious chocolate. The addition of nonfat yogurt instead of whole milk or cream makes it an especially healthy treat.

Ingredients

- 8 ounces brewed coffee, cooled
- ¾ cup plain nonfat yogurt *
- 2 teaspoons brown sugar
- 1 teaspoon chocolate extract
- ½ teaspoon cinnamon, ground
- ½ cup crushed ice or 3 cubes
- Unsweetened cocoa, sprinkle

Directions

Puree all ingredients, except the ice, in a blender until smooth. Gradually add ice and blend until you achieve the frothiness you desire. Pour into tall glasses and sift unsweetened cocoa over the top.

* You can substitute coffee-flavored or chocolate-flavored yogurt for extra richness.

Serves 4 or more

IRISH COFFEE CREAM CORDIAL

I can't claim that this potion offers specific health benefits, but it's a great way to liven up a party and open lines of communication. (See photo on page 46.)

Ingredients

- 1 can (14-ounce) sweetened, condensed milk
- 1 cup strongly brewed coffee, cooled (or 1 cup Irish cream liqueur)
- 1 cup whipping cream
- 4 eggs

Directions

Combine all ingredients in a blender and mix until smooth. I like to serve this cordial straight in small liqueur cups, but if you prefer a less potent but icier potion, pour it over ice-filled highball glasses.

I hope the information and recipes have added to your enjoyment of the exotic potion that coffee represents. To end this section, here's a thought to contemplate over your next cup of joe. The quotation is by Sheik Abd-al-Kadir, sixteenth-century author of *In Praise of Coffee*.

CHICORY

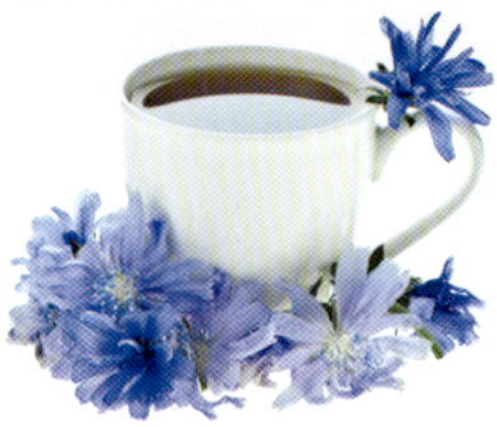

(Cicorium intybus)

If everything I've mentioned about coffee doesn't convince you of its merits, or you know someone who has given up coffee but still thirsts for the aroma and taste, I've a solution: roasted chicory root.

Chicory is an herb that thrives almost anywhere, especially in dry, calcareous soils. Its use as a coffee substitute can be traced back to the Civil War when the Union Army blockaded shipments of coffee to the Confederacy. That's when Southerners took to cutting, roasting, grinding, and brewing the root of the plant that they called "coffee weed." Today the mellow, slightly caramel-flavored taste of coffee mixed with chicory is still enjoyed not only in the South, but worldwide. Luzianne™, a coffee and tea company based in New Orleans, offers this aromatic blend. In the *Language of Flowers* this botanical stands for "frugality." The sobriquet is appropriate because by drinking inexpensive, roasted chicory, a person both economizes and eliminates the caffeine.

Just because the root is the part that goes into making a coffee substitute doesn't mean that the rest of the plant is useless. On the contrary, the pretty little sky-blue flowers open and close at the same time each day, making chicory a valuable addition to a floral clock. Young chicory leaves also lend a slightly bitter, tangy flavor to soups and stews. Eaten fresh in a salad they taste something like Belgian endive, which is a variety of chicory. The root is also a diuretic, laxative, and liver tonic.

According to the *Doctrine of Signatures*, a descriptive system for plants developed in medieval times, chicory is ruled by the planet Uranus. This means that, theoretically, you can add it to potions to cause unusual effects. Legend has it that if you cut the plant with a golden scythe at noon on July 25 and make a drink potion from it, chicory will make you invisible and help you open locked doors and chests. Mark your calendar and let me know if this works. Then again, you'll be invisible to me, so I guess I'll never know!

CHICORY INTUITION ENHANCER

According to folklore, chicory stimulates the intuitive mind, although there is no scientific evidence to support this claim. If you'd like to take a stab at opening your intuitive receptors with a chicory infusion, prepare a cup of chicory or Luzianne according to the directions on the package. Spice it with pinches of anise, clove, and cinnamon, and drink it black. It is hoped that your intuition will blossom like the chicory flower!

What the Wise Beans Have to Say about Your Future

Obviously, the last potion has opened your intuitive receptors and they are now ready to blast off. Why not take advantage of your newly sharpened faculties by learning to read coffee grounds?

The art of interpreting coffee grounds to clarify present situations and predict the future undoubtedly is as ancient as tealeaf reading and the techniques for interpretation are similar.

Other than instant coffee, which dissolves completely in hot water, you can read any kind of grounds. By tradition, the finer, powdery Greek, Turkish, and Arabian brews described above are the most frequently used. If you prefer a coarser grind, put it through a filter and add ½ teaspoon of the filtered remains into the cup so that some sediment is left at the bottom to read after the coffee is drunk.

Items Required

The most convenient kind of vessel to prepare coffee for divination is something called an *Ibrik* or ethnic pot. This traditional Mediterranean coffeepot with a long handle and pointed tip at the rim pours the coffee easily. If you don't want to invest in an *Ibrik*, any small saucepan will do perfectly well.

Some seasoned interpreters prefer to read the grounds from a demitasse cup or in a very small teacup that is solid white on the inside with the rim wider than the base. If you are just getting your feet wet reading the grounds, I suggest you pour the coffee into a regular coffee cup instead of the traditional demitasse-type so that you get clearer and more numerous images.

The saucer is also important in coffee-ground reading because you always read it. You don't want images ingrained in the saucer or cup to interfere with your interpretation, so make sure the saucer's color is solid and that it is undecorated.

Preparations

Many methods to prepare the grounds for reading have come down to us over the ages.

To make Turkish-style coffee for coffee ground reading, boil together 1 teaspoonful of finely ground coffee and one of sugar in 1 cup of water. As soon as the water boils, remove the pot from the heat and stir the contents. Repeat this procedure two more times, stirring until a froth forms. Then pour the unfiltered mixture into a cup. If you use a coffeemaker that removes all of the grounds from the finished product, add a pinch or two of fresh grounds to the full cup so you have enough to read. Coffee grounds stuck between the teeth are definitely not a fashion statement, so let them settle before drinking.

Before your inquirer–the person having the reading, who may be you–takes the first sip, scan the full cup for bubbles that may form to see if they create any recognizable shapes. Perhaps you'll spy a visitor coming, or find that money is on its way. According to one tradition, a single large bubble on top of the coffee stands for disappointing news. In another, a bubble harbingers a friend who will lend a hand in difficult times.

Have your inquirer drink the coffee until only one teaspoonful of liquid remains in the bottom of the cup. Ask the person to stir the grounds, which will include some sugar, until a syrupy consistency forms. Next direct the drinker to swirl the liquid around in the cup three times counterclockwise, and afterwards invert the cup on the saucer. Don't place a napkin on top of the saucer to absorb the liquid because you will eventually also read the saucer.

For the moment, your inquirer will hang onto the cup, keeping it inverted. You pick up the saucer and slowly pour the liquid down the sink drain. Carry the saucer back to the table and ask the inquirer to prop the inverted cup on the side of the saucer to let air flow inside. Coffee grounds should dry out completely before you attempt to read them. Once this happens, reach for the cup, turn it right-side-up, and begin your reading.

If the grounds form a big amorphous clump, either you put in too many or you did not stir them thoroughly. On the other hand, it may mean that your inquirer's life is fraught with confusion. If the grounds look too sparse and light-colored, you probably did not put in enough coffee. In either case, assuming your inquirer can handle more caffeine, you'll need to prepare a second cup.

Interpreting the Grounds

The basic technique for reading coffee grounds was invented by the Turks and refined in South America. In the same way artists study and reinterpret the Old Masters, New Age-style readers and authors to whom this art has been handed down orally, have refined their interpretations by adding details based on their own experiences.

To orient yourself to perform the reading, know that the handle represents the inquirer, the inquirer's immediate environment, and/or present time. Images that appear to be advancing toward the handle show events that may occur in the future; images moving away in the direction of the far side of the cup indicate influences passing out of the inquirer's life.

Coffee Grounds Make Special Patterns

Coffee grounds tend to swirl into a few large, vivid, easily decipherable symbols. In my experience, in order to better distinguish the fine images that take shape in the dried syrup, it helps to soften my vision by squinting.

Magzcha Westerman in *Your Fortune in a Cup* (Trafford Publishing, 2005) confirms my observation that the grounds often adhere into one or two large symbols. She also observes that coffee grounds often stretch out into long, slender, sometimes undulating columns. She interprets the columns as journeys–the longer the column, the more extensive the journey. Other readers maintain that serpentine columns reveal the inquirer's vacillating moods. Straight columns may signify that the inquirer has a clear idea of the path to follow. Here are other special signs that often appear in the coffee cup:

- Dots–movement in a situation. Very small dots refer to words.
- Triangle–an influential man.
- Tripod–an influential woman. If the symbol appears all white in color, she is blonde.
- Crown or teeth-like shape–family.
- Trident–sadness.
- Bubble in the bottom of the cup–the grave.
- Star or flower–in one tradition, they hint at death. In others, a star symbolizes success and a flower stands for love and happiness.
- Numeral 4–money coming to the inquirer soon.

Of Saucers and Thumbprints

Westerman notes that she also reads the grounds left over in the saucer after the excess liquid from the cup has been poured off. She treats the saucer as a separate mini-reading, which in her experience can sometimes reveal the visage of a guardian spirit, angel, or totem animal.

After reading the cup, but before she looks at the saucer, Westerman has her inquirer stick a moistened thumb into the center of the bottom of the cup to make a thumbprint. She instructs the inquirer not to press so hard that a complete white space results, nor so softly that no grounds adhere to the thumb. She comments on the thumbprint pattern left inside the cup with regard to the immediate present or near future.

If you have read tea leaves, you will appreciate that I have tried replicating this technique in tealeaf reading to no avail. The leaves always crumble away or become too lumpy to produce the same clear results of the finely sifted, syrupy coffee leavings. The only kind of tea you might be able to do this with is green Matcha tea, which is fine and powdery.

Curious Divinations for Coffee Abstainers

For inveterate tea drinkers who wouldn't think of letting coffee pass their lips, Sandra Mizumoto Posey has devised some clever, if complex, alternative ways to practice coffee divination. In her book *Café Nation* (Santa Monica Press, 2000), she treats the coffee bean like a rune, shell, bone, or I Ching coin, which are other common forms of geomantic divination (divination using groups of small, like objects from nature).

She has devised a system of prognostication where the inquirer tosses a whole bean onto a flat surface five times. She notes whether the bean lands with the open side or rounded side up. Five throws create a five-pointed star, or pentagram, with thirty-two possible combinations of open and rounded variations. If you are familiar with African/Brazilian cowrie shell divination, the idea is similar. Posey has penned meanings for these variations, which are reminiscent of the explanations found in the ancient I Ching's *Book of Changes*. Each star belongs to a suit that carries a unique significance. She has also put together a spin-off on the I Ching yarrow stick divination that uses wooden coffee stirrers and a pentagram system as opposed to the hexagrams of the I Ching. In my opinion, although this may seem a complicated method to predict your future, it makes a green way to recycle all of those wooden coffee stirrers.

So far, we've journeyed through the wonderful worlds of tea and coffee as supreme potion ingredients. One might suppose there's nothing left to say.

"But wait," you protest, "What about chocolate, my favorite food?"

Never fear. In the next chapter, I'll take up the marvels of chocolate, corn (yes, you can drink corn), beer, sweeteners, herbal tisanes, and a variety of spices guaranteed to put zing into any potion you aim to create.

Chapter 6

CHOCOLATE, BEER & SUGAR

Who Could Ask for Anything More?

More, indeed. This chapter focuses on the best of the rest of potion-crafting ingredients. Naturally, we begin with many people's idea of the very best food: chocolate.

Chocolate: Food of the Gods

A Spoonful of Chocolate History

This divine drink builds up resistance and fights fatigue. A cup of this precious drink permits a man to walk for an entire day without food.
–Hernán Cortés (1485–1547)
Spanish Conquistador of Mexico

When the conquistadors arrived in Mexico, the emperor Moctezuma offered his guests steaming bowlfuls of a mysterious, thick, dark-brown liquid. The Aztecs called their highly aromatic, intensely flavored substance the Food of the Gods. We call it chocolate.

Mesoamerican cultures celebrated with this drink during important life events such as baptism and marriage. They believed that chocolate was such a vital source of knowledge and wisdom that they sometimes substituted it for blood in their rituals. Perhaps this was how Alfred Hitchcock got the idea to use chocolate instead of ketchup in the blood-curdling shower scene of the black-and-white film *Psycho*... Cocoa beans were so prized among the Aztecs that they used them for currency. Four beans could buy a turkey and 100 could buy a slave.

The politically incorrect term "redskin" actually originated with the Maya Indians. They slathered a reddish-colored paste on their bodies made from the outer coating of crushed cacao and annatto seeds. The paste protected their skin from the intense tropical sun's rays, thereby creating the first suntan lotion. Today you can still mix unsweetened cocoa with heavy cream and olive oil for a super moisturizing facial masque.

Chocolate's Cradle

Chocolate is extracted from the seed (known as a bean) of the cacao tree, native to tropical regions of Mexico, Central and South America. The forty-foot evergreen blossoms with fragrant clusters of creamy white and pink flowers.

The flowers mature into little football-shaped fruit that looks something like ribbed, pointed melons. As the fruit matures, it changes color to yellow, orange, and even purplish red, making the tree appear to be decked out for Christmas. Inside the fruit's pulp, the little cacao beans arrange themselves in a column around a pinkish core.

After the beans are harvested, they are fermented to intensify the flavor. Then they are dried, cleaned, and roasted, and the shells removed. During the processing, the beans are ground into a liquefied cocoa mass. Approximately half of this mass consists of a fat called cocoa butter. When separated from the rest, this buttery substance emits a pleasant, chocolaty odor that never turns rancid. Cocoa butter can be made into a face or body cream, soap, or talcum powder. The remaining fat-free substance is called a cocoa solid.

Nutritional Power of Chocolate

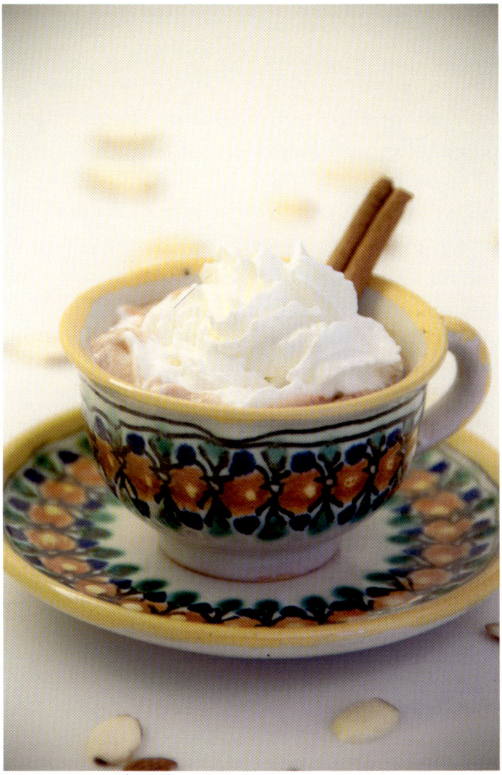

Mexican Hot Chocolate. **(Recipe on page 63.)**

The Aztecs considered chocolate an aphrodisiac. Turns out they weren't far off the mark in their empirical observations. Laboratory studies have since shown that cacao contains a chemical (phenyl ethylamine) that causes the brain to think it's falling in love.

Chocolate packs a lot of energy. In fact, a person can walk 150 steps on the energy provided by a single chocolate chip. At the same time this substance has the ability to calm the emotions. In fact, consuming dark chocolate can lower blood pressure and get rid of both a headache and constipation (the latter when mixed with cayenne.) It is also high in potassium, an essential mineral. Brushing your teeth with chocolate-infused toothpaste has been proven to strengthen tooth enamel. What an incentive for your child to brush!

Chocolate's caffeine content is low compared to coffee or even tea. Here's what the USDA National Nutrient Database has to say about milligrams of caffeine in different types of chocolate. For comparisons with tea and coffee, see those entries.

Item	Amount	Caffeine Content
Baking chocolate, unsweetened	1 ounce	25 mg
Semi-sweet chocolate	1 ounce	13 mg
Chocolate chips	¼ cup	13 mg
Milk chocolate bar	4 ounces	3-to-10 mg
White chocolate bar	4 ounces	2-to-4 mg
Dark chocolate bar	4 ounces	28 mg
Chocolate milk	8 ounces	8 mg
Chocolate mousse from Jell-O® mix	½ cup	6 mg
Chocolate covered espresso bean	1	3-to-5 mg
Chocolate powder mix	3 heaping teaspoons	8 mg
Chocolate syrup	2 tablespoons	5 mg
Hot cocoa mix	1 envelope	5 mg

Evolution of Chocolate

Chocolate was not always the sweet treat we think of today. The first European settlers in the Americas were underwhelmed by its bitter taste. As time passed, colonists in the West Indies hit on the idea to pour hot chocolate directly from the pot into an enormous dish or basin that contained sugar, another indigenous crop. People sat around the basin and drank from it with dippers. And so, the first chocolate lovers were born. Chocolate Houses, similar to today's cafés, were established in London beginning in 1657. The drink remained a luxury beverage until well into the nineteenth century.

Chocolate Comes into Its Own

Improving chocolate was a multicultural effort. First, the Spaniards introduced pinches of cinnamon into the brew. They also liked to froth their hot chocolate with a special stick still used in Spanish-speaking countries today. Then the French made their mark by adding milk. The English experimented with leaving some cocoa butter in the solids, which resulted in solid chocolate. The inventive Dutch discovered a method to wash cocoa in an alkali solution so that it dissolved more easily in water; hence the term "Dutch Chocolate."

Finally, the Swiss invented a machine that eliminated the graininess. They also invented milk chocolate by adding condensed milk to the mix. Today over ninety percent of the chocolate consumed in the US is milk chocolate, although dark chocolate is making inroads due to its touted health benefits.

Besides dark and semi-sweet chocolate, which contain no milk and milk chocolate, there's baking chocolate. This kind consists of cocoa solids and cocoa butter, but no sugar. White chocolate, made from cocoa butter, milk, and sugar, does not contain cocoa solids.

Like Tea for Chocolate?

Lately, chocolate combined with tea has become a chic trend with hundreds of variations now available on gourmet tea shop shelves. The concept was born in nineteenth century France. Sometime during the middle of that century, the Mariage Frères brothers inherited their father's tea importation business. As the younger generation often does, they decided to improve the business by creating their own tea blends. One of their ideas was to blend two popular ingredients, tea and chocolate. The result was the famous *Chocolat des Mandarins*. Together the brothers invented more than 200 tea blends, most of which can still be purchased today. As far as potion-crafting is concerned, the tea uplifts the full-bodied flavor of the chocolate.

Word of Advice for Potion-Crafters

When rustling up potions, remember that cocoa is darker in color and less sweet and fatty than chocolate. Although it is easier to mix with other liquids, it does not exude the same fine flavor as chocolate. Mexicans mix chocolate with chili powder to perk up a sauce called *mole* that they pour over enchiladas and other main dishes. I'm sure I don't need to tell you that chocolate is also a main ingredient in many desserts as well as the liqueur *crème de cacao.* Read on for two of my favorite liquid chocolate potions.

Serves 6

MEXICAN HOT CHOCOLATE

When I lived in Mexico City as a foreign exchange student, my host family went out of their way to dazzle me every day with local culinary delights. One of my favorites was the way they prepared hot chocolate. Many a cool, damp night was spent with the entire family of ten cozied around the electric fire in the breakfast room, sipping the hot, frothy brew and exchanging the day's news. I want to share my host family's recipe here so that you, too, may incorporate this warm and friendly tradition in your own home.

Ingredients

- ¼ cup unsweetened cocoa
- ½ cup sugar
- 1 tablespoon almonds, ground
- 1 teaspoon cinnamon, ground
- Dash salt
- 1 quart milk
- ¼ cup light cream
- 1 teaspoon vanilla extract

Directions

In a small bowl, combine the cocoa, sugar, almonds, cinnamon, and salt. Mix well, and set aside. In a medium saucepan, heat the milk until it bubbles; lower the heat. Stir in the dry ingredients and beat with a rotary beater until smooth. Stirring constantly, return the saucepan to boiling. Add the cream and vanilla and heat gently. Before serving, stir the cocoa once more with rotary beater until frothy. Pour into mugs and garnish with a sprinkling of ground cinnamon or insert one cinnamon stick in each cup.

Serves 1

Sagacious CHOCOLATE SAUCE

Photograph by C. Nathan Pulley Photography

Can anything as sinfully delicious as chocolate also help you obtain wisdom? The Maya people believed that eating chocolate aided meditation and brought a person closer to the All-One. Who am I to disagree with ancient Maya perspicacity?

To that end, here's an ice cream topper recipe that is out of this world. Pour it over apple or almond ice cream, as both of these botanicals are thought to confer insight and understanding. If you use vanilla ice cream, the vanilla will help you gain peace of mind. Pour the sauce over cinnamon ice cream and you may improve your memory.

Alas, this recipe is not for those watching their weight, but it is oh, so good! And a dollop of delight (and wisdom) can't possibly interfere *too* much with your diet.

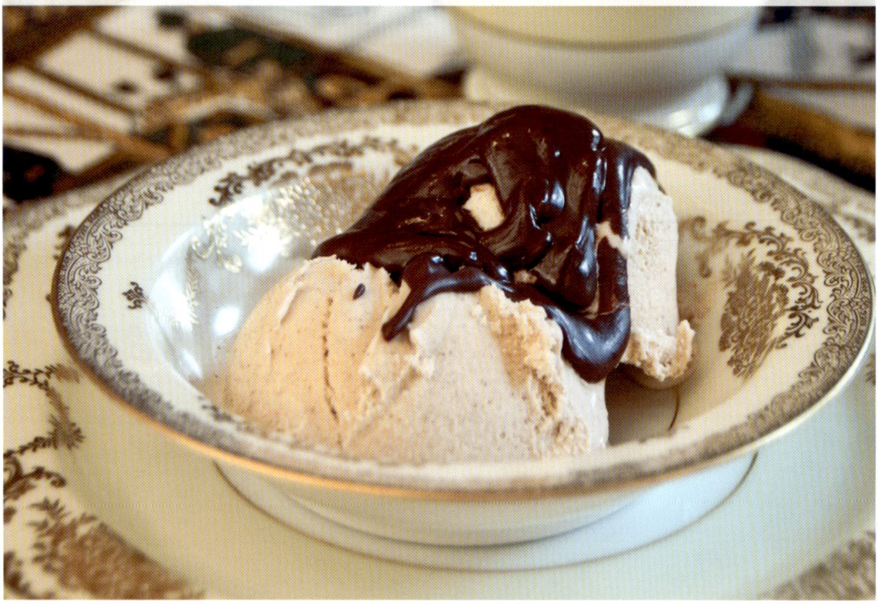

Ingredients

- ¾ cup whipping cream
- ½ cup butter
- ¼ cup sugar
- 6 ounces unsweetened chocolate, broken into small pieces
- 2 tablespoons water (If you prefer an alcoholic potion, substitute crème de cacao.)

Directions

Heat the cream with the butter and sugar in the top pot of a double boiler. Stir until smooth. Beat in the chocolate until melted. Add water a little at a time, blending until smooth. Pour over the ice cream and serve.

OTHER BOTANICALS ALLEGED TO CONFER KNOWLEDGE AND WISDOM INCLUDE

Cinquefoil	Bay	Sage
Solomon's seal	Olive	Corn

Valuable Potion Ingredients

In this section, I'd like to highlight some ingredients to enliven your potions. They include beer, onions, garlic, olives, salt, sweeteners, spices, and even that well-known but underrated American standby, ketchup. Let's begin with a common vegetable that most people are accustomed to eating rather than drinking: corn.

CORN

(Latin Name: Zea Mays)

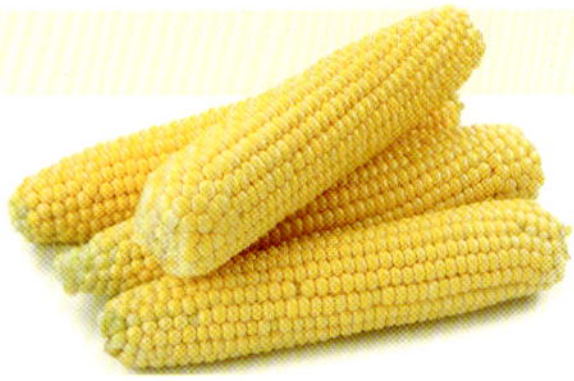

Every summer tall cornstalks ripple in green waves across the fields of the Great Plains. The sweet, chewy grain shucked from the cobs comes in a variety of colors from yellow and white to blue, purple, and even dark red. Corn originated in the Americas and is a staple grain of many Native cultures.

All parts of the corn are valuable in herbal medicine. For example, cornstarch, which is derived from corn, can be used as a facial cleanser instead of soap, and the cornstalks added to the bath help soften skin. Eating the kernels lowers cholesterol. Corn silk tea promotes kidney functioning and corn cob tea reduces swelling of the wrists, ankles, and abdomen. Some culinary uses of corn include popcorn, cornmeal, cornstarch, corn syrup, corn oil, hominy grits, and corn flour used for baking bread, cakes, and tortillas.

Like all sustaining grains, corn has many uses in potion-crafting. However, I notice that some authors mistakenly write about corn lore as originating in European cultures. Unfortunately, those writers misinterpret documents that use the term "corn" to refer to any number of other grains. Corn is a product of the New World. It was not farmed in the Old World until it was brought back from Mexico during the sixteenth century. Until recently in Europe, corn has been cultivated mostly to feed livestock.

In Mesoamerica corn was sacred to the Corn Mother and Father. This grain represented the great cycles of life because the Maya year was based on the cycle of corn cultivation. Therefore, corn can be included in potions to discover information about personal, community, regional, and even the Earth's cycles.

OLIVE

(Latin Name: Olea europaea)

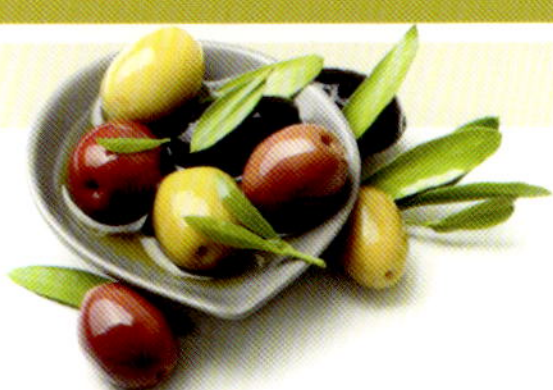

Olives were so basic to the daily meals of ancient Mediterranean cultures that those people offered the fruit to their gods. Modern science has shown that olive oil promotes healthy HDL cholesterol levels. Olives make a welcome addition to sauces, fish, game, and meat dishes.

In former times, olive oil was used as the base for many anointing oils because it was thought to concentrate the authority of kings and priests. It was also alleged to cure drunkenness and deliver a person or animal from enchantment. In the *Language of Flowers* olives stand for "peace," and so have come to be associated with tranquility and spirituality. Add the oil to potions, especially sauces, to gain wisdom and increase your powers of concentration.

Serves 6-12

Flor Crawford's
CHICHA MORADA

One variety of purple corn native to Peru is made into a deliciously refreshing grapelike-tasting beverage called *Chicha Morada*. This drink has been enjoyed for centuries–perhaps millennia. To produce it, Peruvians boil purple corn together with pineapple, and sometimes apple and/or quince fruit, and add cinnamon and clove for spice.

Purple corn, besides tasting good, is distinguished for its nutritional attributes. It contains anthocyanin, a class of flavonoid that acts as an antioxidant that is more powerful than blueberries. Anthocyanin also slows the degeneration of internal organs and the skin, promotes healing, and helps prevent cardiovascular disease. No wonder so many Peruvians of Native descent live to a ripe old age.

Thanks to the influence of Latino immigrants, you can now buy bottled *Chicha Morada* at Latin food markets. It is also sold powdered like Jell-O so that all you need do is add juices of pineapple, lemon, lime, and apple.

If you can find dried purple corn kernels and would like to try making it from scratch, here's a recipe offered by my very good Peruvian friend Flor Crawford. She introduced me to *Chicha Morada* when we went to Peru together on an intercultural training assignment. I found the drink to be quite reviving after a long day's work.

Ingredients

- 1-2 liters water
- 1-2 pounds dried purple corn kernels, washed
- 1-2 apples, peels only
- Peels of 1 pineapple
- 3 cloves, whole
- 3-6 6-inch cinnamon sticks
- Juice of 1-2 lemons
- Sugar to taste

Directions

Put the water in a pot, add the purple corn, apple and pineapple peels, cloves, and cinnamon. Cover and bring to a boil; reduce heat and simmer for approximately 1 hour. Use a colander to strain the liquid and let the mixture cool. Only prepare the amount that you are going to consume right away. Before serving, add the lemon juice, sugar, some shredded apple, and very small pieces of pineapple and stir everything together. Serve in tall glasses.

BEER

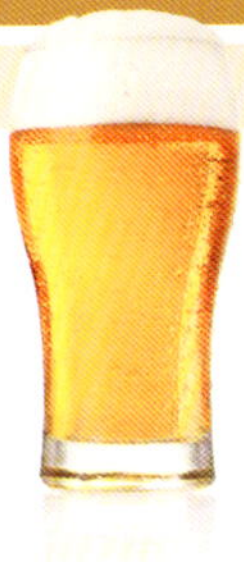

(Latin Name: Cerevisia)

You may be accustomed to adding wine to potions, especially in punches and sauces, but many of us don't think to add beer. The Latin name of this favorite pub and bar beverage is derived from the Greek goddess Ceres, Lady of the Harvest of Grain.

Beer can be brewed from just about any fermented grain, including barley, corn, rice, and wheat. Almost all beers are flavored with hops, which were originally added to retard spoilage. Hops, which you can purchase at an herb store, can be drunk on its own as an infusion or blended with other botanicals, such as chamomile and valerian to promote restful sleep. A grain-based, alcoholic beverage without hops flavoring is called ale.

Without a doubt, beer has amazing nutritional value. It raises levels of good HDL cholesterol and helps keep blood from clotting, which is important to stave off heart attack and stroke. Drinking beer lowers the risk of developing kidney stones–probably because of the high water content. This beverage also keeps a person from falling prey to several cancers and the silicon in it stimulates bone growth. Pour flat beer on your hair while you're conditioning it in the shower to add volume and shine.

As happens with overindulgence in any form of alcohol, drinking more than two 12-ounce beers per day for men and one for women can lead to liver damage, heart problems, breast cancer, gout, and more. Not to mention the calories, which weigh in at 150 for a regular 12-ounce bottle of beer and around 100 for the lighter versions.

Beer is mostly an ingredient of Northern European cuisine as wine is in Southern Europe. The difference is that beer's flavor succeeds in a more limited range of dishes. For liquid potions, add beer to beef sauces, stews, and cheese fondues. As to potion-crafting, beer is thought to help bring ideas and projects to fruition.

GARLIC

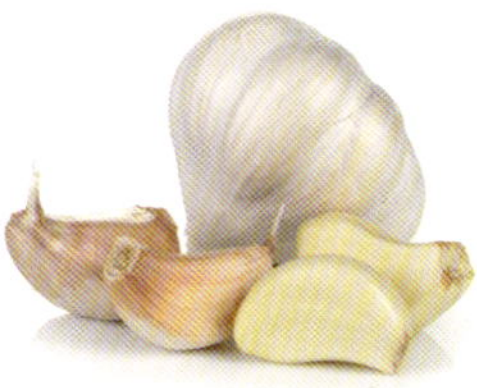

(Latin Name: Allium sativum)

It may come as a surprise that this plant with its pungent-smelling bulb is actually a member of the delicately fragrant lily family. The cloves that comprise the bulb are packed with vitamins A, B-1 (thiamine), B-2 (riboflavin), and C, so natural food buffs look on garlic as something of a panacea. It has been touted to help cure everything from the common cold to coughs, sore throats, fungus infections, intestinal disorders, rheumatism, herpes, and even snakebite. Garlic has been experimented with as an agent to help stamp out the polio and HIV viruses. The juice pressed from the bulb is proven to lower blood pressure and bad cholesterol levels as well as prevent heart attack.

Garlic is famous for the strong but irresistible flavor it imparts to many ethnic dishes. Cooking it, however, makes it lose much of its garlicky flavor along with many of the nutrients. When buying garlic, avoid shriveled or dried up bulbs. Store bulbs in a cool, dark place such as a ventilated bag or in a vegetable basket. When adding it to juice, 1 or 2 cloves suffice. If you juice a leafy green vegetable along with the garlic, fold the clove inside the leaf before slipping it into the juicer to keep from contaminating the sides of the container with the overpowering flavor.

Ancient Egyptians and Romans extolled the physical and psychological virtues of garlic, and believed that it granted them strength, courage, and longevity. This mighty bulb is renowned in folklore from ancient to modern times for its ability to protect against evil, especially vampires (as is attested by Hollywood horror movies), ghosts, poltergeists, and the plague. It is perfectly possible that at least in the case of the plague, this myth may contain a bulb of truth. Fleas, including the plague-carrying kind, tend to shun garlic-exuding skin for tastier meals.

In modern times, garlic is added to potions to clear the mind and render a person better able to make good choices and judgments. Recent studies on the psychology of scent show that garlic can actually be a turn-on. So it follows that the plant may be used as a love potion ingredient. Bring on the garlic soup!

ONION

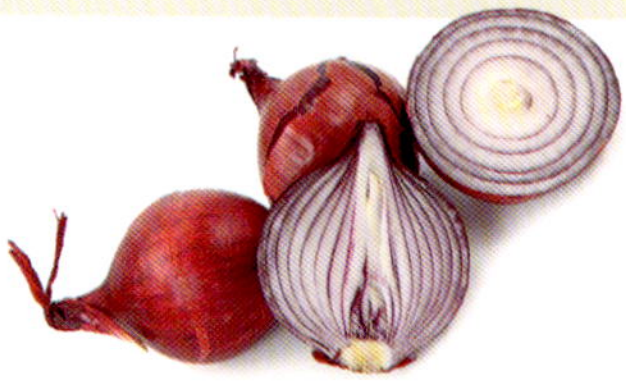

(Latin Name: Allium)

Like garlic, this yellow, white, or red bulb is member of the lily family. I prefer to grow my own or buy organic onions cultivated without pesticides, and always choose ones without cuts, blemishes, or patchy fungus. Store your bulbs in a cool, dry place such as a root cellar, but do not refrigerate.

At 55 calories per average-size bulb, onions make an ideal choice for dieters. They are loaded with vitamins B, C, and K, and calcium. Onions promote good blood circulation and help dissolve clots. If you can stand eating half an onion per day you will raise your good HDL cholesterol level by 30 percent. Then again, you may risk chasing away your friends with the strong odor.

Onion juice tastes as strong as garlic, but you can sweeten it in your potions with apple juice. To my taste buds, white onions have the mildest flavor, yet they seem to keep less well than the yellow and red varieties. If you can't stand the oniony intensity in your potion, try substituting milder-flavored chives, leeks, or shallots.

Ancient astrologers linked the onion to the planet Mars and Fire element. Alexander the Great believed that if his troops ate onions, their aggressive tendencies would increase. Conversely, in India eating onions is supposed to have a tranquilizing effect. Potions concocted from onion juice are alleged to excite sexual desire, instill a person with self-confidence, enhance intuition, and ensure success. Because the onion bulb grows in rings, it represents life's cycles, and can be consumed in potions to celebrate births, deaths, or any of life's transitions.

SALT

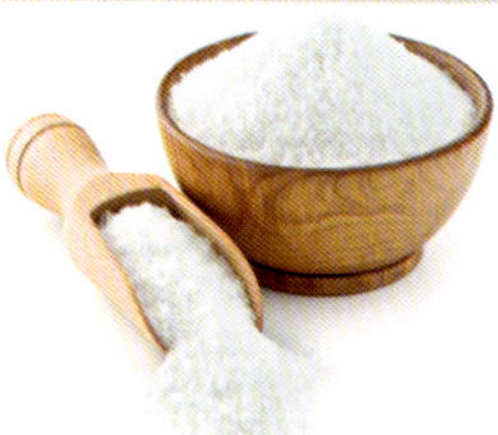

(Sodium Chloride)

Salt is a vital mineral for both humans and animals. Our blood contains a lot of salt; without it, we could not live. Before refrigeration and canning were invented, salt was our primary way to preserve food. We make what we eat and drink taste better by adding it to our food.

We take in approximately 2,000 milligrams of salt per day in our food. The problem is that as a culture, we consume so much salt that it can adversely affect blood pressure, heart, kidneys, bones, and hormone and electrolyte balance. To help protect your health, the recipes in this book include minimal amounts of salt.

In myth, salt was sacred to Osiris and Set of the Egyptian pantheon and to the sea gods Poseidon and Neptune. As you learned in Chapter 3, you can use salt in potion-crafting to cleanse and purify your body, potion-crafting tools, and your kitchen. Place several grains in a dish on your desk or wherever you work to aid concentration.

KETCHUP

(Also spelled "Catsup")

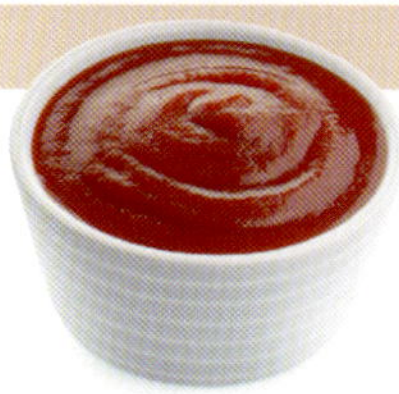

Notice how I sneaked in this ingredient at the end of this section out of alphabetical order. I imagine that the last additive you were expecting to see in a healthy potions book is ketchup. Yet, as a kind of sauce, it deserves mention. Ketchup is defined as any salty extract of fish, shellfish, and vegetables, including mushrooms, usually in a tomato base.

There are those, including famous chefs, who won't tolerate ketchup in their restaurants because they think it's some sort of American abomination. Actually, ketchup was not invented in the US, although the Heinz and Hunts companies have popularized it here. The original ketchup, which did not include tomatoes, was invented in China. It was called *ke-tsiap*, which in the Amoy dialect means "brine." This sauce was composed of fish brine, kidney beans, anchovies, mushrooms, and walnuts. The recipe traveled to Indonesia and Malaysia, where British sailors took it back to England. There people pickled anchovies and oysters in it. Tomatoes didn't enter into the mix until the 1700s after this fruit was discovered in Latin America.

Today's typical ketchup is made from tomato concentrate, plus allspice, celery, cinnamon, garlic, salt, and sugar or corn syrup. Innovations currently unfolding in the wild world of ketchup just might take those snobs who abhor the sauce by surprise. In a recent *New York Times* interview with José Andrés and Thomas Keller of American Eats Tavern in Washington, DC, these chefs make it clear that designer ketchups are catching on. At their restaurant they serve over a dozen different gourmet ketchups from blueberry to mushroom, red currant, yellow tomato, cherry, oyster, anchovy, spiceberry, and more. On the West Coast Angelinos are scarfing up such exotic ketchups as ginger, jalapeño, whole spice, mustard, and fig.

I doubt whether ketchup exfoliates the skin as the character in the quotation claims. But since all of the above listed ingredients are considered aphrodisiacs, feel free to experiment with making your own ketchup potion. Then pour the sauce over your food to stimulate ardor.

Sweet Dreams Are Made of This: About Sweeteners

Many potions taste best when sweetened, so in this section we'll take a look at sweeteners. Sugar beets and sugar cane provide most of the sugar we consume. Cane sugar is one of the oldest forms of sugar, having been cultivated in South and East Asia since at least 1000 BCE. Europeans only started using it after the Middle Ages. Up to then, they relied mostly on honey, corn, fruits (such as grapes), malt, maple, milk, and sorghum grass. Many tropical cultures also derived sweeteners from coconuts.

Typically, highly refined granulated (white) sugar is a basic potion ingredient. In processing this sugar, the molasses, which contains all of the nutrition, is washed away. What remains is pure carbohydrate. This makes your potion taste good and provides energy in the form of calories. As with salt, the American diet includes too much sugar. We add 320–350 calories to our daily diets from this substance. High sugar consumption contributes to such health problems as allergies, hyperactivity in children, diabetes, eczema, osteoporosis, high LDL cholesterol levels, vaginal yeast infections, and lowered resistance to bacterial infections.

While I'm not advocating you eliminate sugar from your diet, and several recipes in this book include it as an ingredient, the lighter you go on this sweetener, the better it will be for your health. When you do use sugar, I

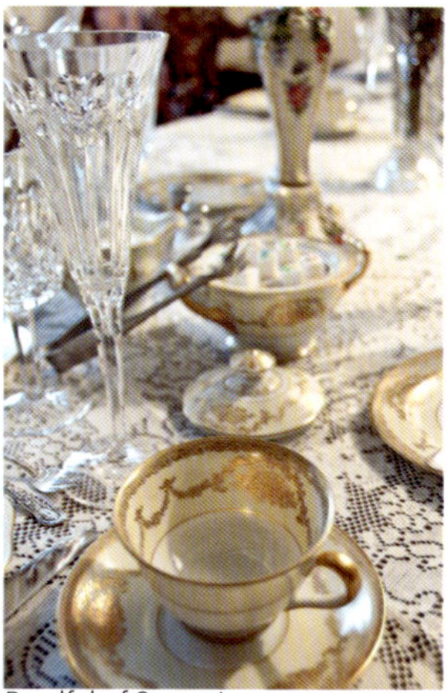

Photograph by C. Nathan Pulley Photography

Bowlful of Sugar. Lump sugar dissolves easily in hot liquid and is oh-so pretty.

recommend that you buy organic. Even the big supermarket chains now carry reasonably inexpensive house brands of organic sugar. If you would like to learn more about how to decrease sugar in cooking, I recommend the book *Comfort Food Fix: Feel Good Favorites Made Healthy* by Ellie Krieger (Wiley, 2011).

You might also enjoy experimenting with different types of sugar than the refined granulated kind. For example, extra granulated sugar, sometimes called "superfine" or "castor" sugar, dissolves readily in iced drinks. Demerara sugar, which is comprised of large, golden crystals, is a favorite additive for teas and coffees because it dissolves quickly in hot liquid and has a slightly nutty flavor. One of my favorites is called "turbinado." With this semi-raw sugar, the molasses is only partially washed off, which adds a rich taste and nutrients to a potion.

Sugars that do not mix well in liquid potions include confectioners, a type of sugar that is mixed with cornstarch. This type is often used to make frosting. Unlike turbinado, brown sugar is refined sugar that has had some of the molasses sprayed back on. Brown sugar usually does not combine well in liquid potions.

Following are sweeteners other than sugar that you may want to try.

FRUIT, FLOWERS, AND HERBS

As you will learn in Part III, various fruits contain a fair amount of natural sugar. The sweetness is enhanced when combined with other naturally sweet substances, such as milk. When I frequent *Vitaminas* bars in Brazil, I often ask the barista to omit the sugar from my drinks because they are sweet enough on their own.

Although fruit won't work for all of your potions, such as savory soups and sauces, many do. Examples include berries, such as blueberry, raspberry, strawberry, cherry, peach, apple, pear, plum, and dried citrus peel. And don't forget hibiscus and honeysuckle flowers, cinnamon, and licorice.

AGAVE NECTAR

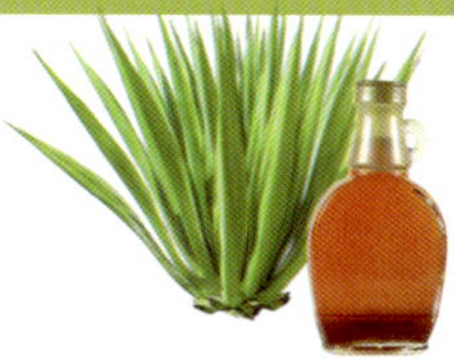

Neither can I recommend agave. Sweet agave nectar extracted from the core of the blue agave succulent has become a recent favorite among health gurus. I know I may make a few enemies here, but I have to say that agave nectar is arguably worse for you than processed sugar. Agave promoters point to the nectar's fairly low glycemic index, meaning that consuming it will not raise your blood sugar levels. However, the reason for this is that agave is very high in fructose, higher even than corn syrup, and cannot be easily metabolized. Overconsumption can lead to fatty liver disease, diabetes, heart disease, and ultimately cancer. It also contains a lot of calories. I'm sure none of us want that.

HONEY

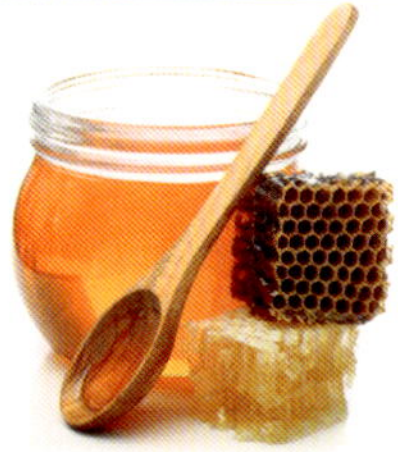

Speaking of honey, this sticky but ethereally fragrant substance has been a favorite sweetener probably ever since the first human worked up the nerve to thrust a hand into a hive. Honey comes in a palette of colors besides yellow, depending on which flowers the bees have visited. It can be white, brown, orange, green, purple–even black–thick or thin, strong or mild. Flavors are equally diverse. Varieties include honey made from eucalyptus, orange blossoms, raspberry, rosemary, sage, and my personal favorite, heather.

Honey contains as much glucose and fructose as sugar, but is less processed, so if you sweeten your potions with honey, you more or less come out a winner. On a recent *Dr. Oz* program, the doctor notes that you should try to buy organic honey. It is thicker and darker, and includes more nutrients.

Because of the way its mild flavor melds seamlessly into a variety of dishes, clover honey is one of the best for potion-crafting. And miracle of miracles, it is one of the cheapest and most readily available kinds! Honey can't always replace sugar because of its viscid consistency, but it is worth taking time to experiment. Some of my smoothie recipes in Part II use honey instead of sugar. Add both sugar and honey to potions for love, happiness, prosperity, good health, and harmony. The following recipe will get you started.

Makes 3-4 glasses

BANANA HONEY SMOOTHIE

Tofu adds a rich and silky touch to this sweet honey and banana smoothie, and an extra nutritional kick, too.

Ingredients

- 2 ripe bananas
- 16 ounces soft tofu, drained
- ½ cup ice, crushed
- 3 tablespoons honey
- ½ teaspoon vanilla extract

Directions

Peel the bananas, cut them into small pieces, and place them in a blender. Cube the tofu and add it, along with the rest of the ingredients. Cover and blend until smooth.

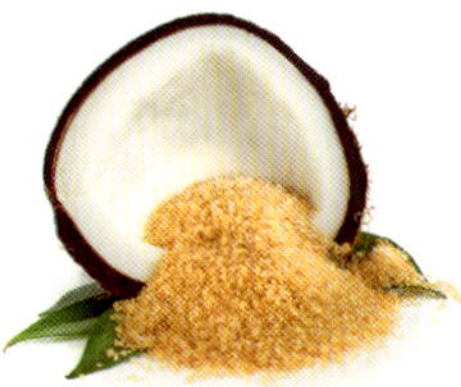

Coconut sugar comes from tapping the sap of the coconut palm tree. It tastes somewhat like brown sugar and dissolves readily in liquids. Although composed of sucrose, this sugar has a lower glycemic index than refined cane or beet sugar. Coconut sugar has been gaining popularity with the health conscious because it is chock full of B vitamins, iron, magnesium, potassium, and zinc, as well as sixteen amino acids. So why am I, a coconut lover, not enthusiastic about replacing refined sugar with coconut sugar?

Simply because I am a coconut lover. Once you tap the trunk of a coconut producing tree and extract the sap, it will no longer produce coconuts. You can reverse this appalling consequence by every three years alternating between growing coconuts and extracting the sap. However, during the coconut producing cycle, the palm will not produce as well nor will the fruit render as many vitamins and minerals. Since lately the demand for various coconut products has been so high, more and more coconut palms are being destroyed. For these reasons, I can't recommend coconut as a sugar substitute.

What to Substitute?

Molasses and maple sugar taste good and are good for you, but they impart a strong, distinctive flavor to potions. You may not want to include this taste in every potion, especially tea. So why not give stevia a try?

STEVIA

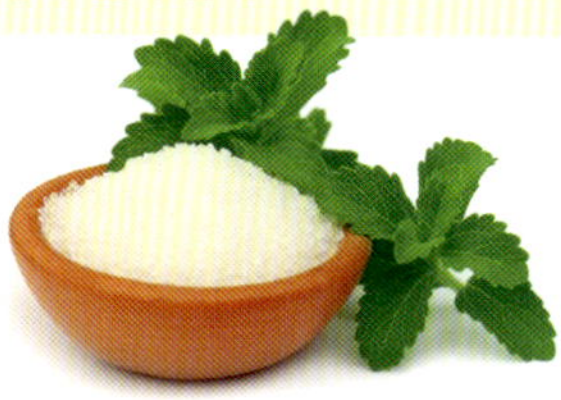

Stevia rebaudiana, also known as sweet leaf, is extracted from the leaves of an herb native to Paraguay and Brazil. This mighty little leaf is 150–400 times sweeter than sugar (claims vary). It contains no calories and has a zero glycemic index.

You may not have heard of stevia until recently. For a long time the non-nutritional sweeteners lobbyists kept it off the US market by persuading the FDA to ban the competition. (Sounds like politics in Washington as usual, doesn't it?) Once the European Union approved this natural sweetener as a sugar substitute, the US felt obliged to certify it, too. The leaf is dried and ground to a powder to use like table sugar.

Stevia is still grown in Paraguay, Uruguay, and Brazil, but has expanded to Japan and California in the US, as well as other countries. You can even grow your own from seed as I did, or buy a plant at your gardening center. If you live in a cold climate, you will have to bring the plant indoors before the first frost.

Stevia may sound like a miracle sugar replacement, but many consumers have not managed to cozy up to it, and for good reason. Although the leaf tastes sweet initially, its lingering bitter flavor fails to satisfy some. A friend of mine discovered this when she chomped on one of the leaves from my plant. In cooking and potion-crafting stevia can turn some dishes an unappetizing brown color. Websites like www.stevia.com show conversion charts for potion-crafting and cooking.

The food industry, however, understands it's latched on to a good thing with sweet leaf. They are constantly experimenting to create brands more suitable to the palette. Look for stevia to become more predominant in the future.

Seven Spices from Your Cupboard to Jazz up Your Potions

I've just discussed sugar, so surely it makes sense to continue with "spice, and everything nice." Following are descriptions of seven extra ingredients to spice up your potions. Why seven instead of six or twelve? When sailors in past centuries explored the seven seas, they brought back exotic seasonings mostly from tropical regions that soon infused into Western cuisine. The following entries, with the exception of mustard, hail from these alluring lands.

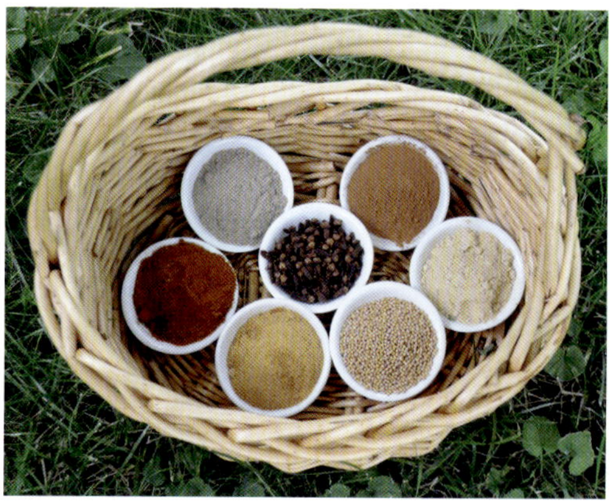

Photograph by C. Nathan Pulley Photography

Seven Spices. Photo shows Cardamom, Cayenne, Cinnamon, Clove, Ginger, Mustard, and Nutmeg.

CARDAMOM

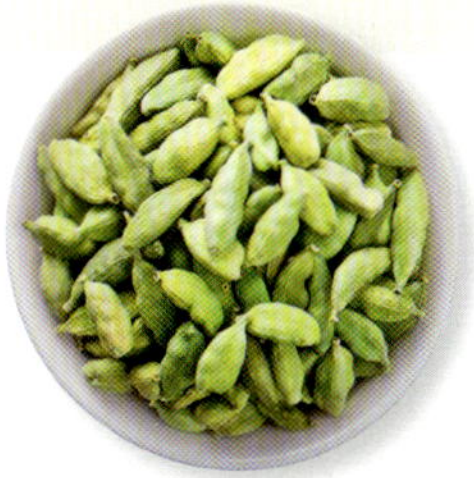

(Latin Name: *Elettaria cardamomum*)

The fragrantly piquant, reddish-brown seeds of this bushy perennial of Middle Eastern origin have been used in perfumery and cooking since ancient times. With the discovery of coffee, the ground seed became a favored flavoring for this drink and is still popular in those countries. These days, the palm-like bush is also cultivated in the West Indies and Central America. Cardamom lends its peppery note to hot milk, Chai, liqueurs, mulled wines, custard, and bread. A little of the ground cardamom seed goes a long way, for it is a purgative in large doses.

Like most spices, cardamom is renowned as an aphrodisiac and fertility booster. People also drink potions with cardamom in the hope of obtaining money, luck, and protection, and to improve general conditions. This botanical is also said to confer happiness and peace of mind and brighten the disposition.

CAYENNE

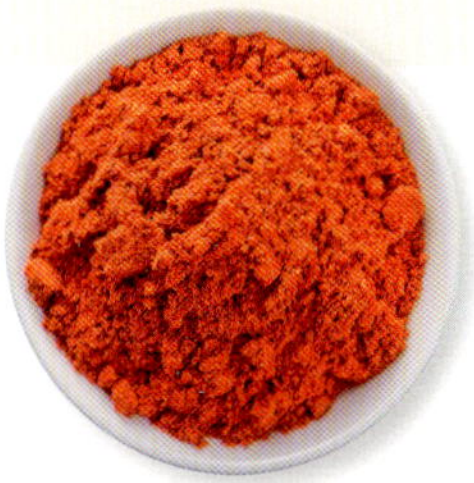

(Latin Name: *Capsicum minimum*)

The name for this hot pepper originates in a Greek word meaning "to bite," so, it should come as no surprise that cayenne is best known as a condiment for hot and spicy Mexican, Mediterranean, and Indian food. As with all peppery seasonings, small amounts stimulate the metabolism for weight loss. Cayenne's antibacterial properties help prevent diarrhea and increase blood circulation. This pepper certainly adds pizzazz to potions, but make sure not to overwhelm the nuances of your brew by adding too much. A mere pinch will activate your potions, and if superstition is to be believed, increase your sex drive, too.

CINNAMON

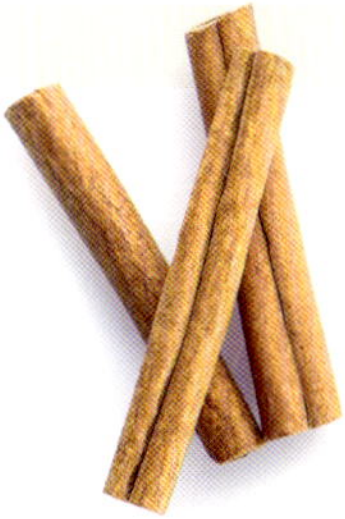

(Latin Name: *Cinnamomum zeylanicum; C. cassia*)

You probably recognize cinnamon as those spicy little sticks frequently used to stir hot apple cider, cocoa, and coffee specialties. The sticks are actually the dried inner bark of a medium-sized laurel tree, native to Sri Lanka. So-called "real" cinnamon comes from the *zeylanicum* tree, but most of the cinnamon available today is harvested from the *cassia* tree. Although gourmet cooks may disagree about the quality, in potion-crafting it doesn't make much difference which kind you use, and cassia is cheaper.

The essential oil comprised part of ancient Egyptian embalming and anointing oils, and at one time was considered more valuable than gold. Today, it is used widely in cookery, perfumery, and incense-making. Usually used in its ground form, cinnamon adds zest to desserts, curries, and some soups. A British friend of mine once commented that when she visits the US, she can smell cinnamon wafting from restaurants and bakeries everywhere. She thinks Americans consume much more cinnamon than the British. Possibly true.

Cinnamon is an antiseptic and astringent. Naturopathic healers use it to ease lower back pain, flatulence, vomiting, and diarrhea. Because essential oil of cinnamon can burn the skin and cause severe eye irritation, you should handle it with care.

In folklore, this bark, like most spices, is touted as an aphrodisiac. At the same time, the energy cinnamon imparts is of a peaceful nature, so it makes an excellent potion with which to bless a room or create a happy home. Cinnamon is also an ingredient of money-draw potions and potions for intuitive self-development, inspiration, improved memory, knowledge, and wisdom.

CLOVE

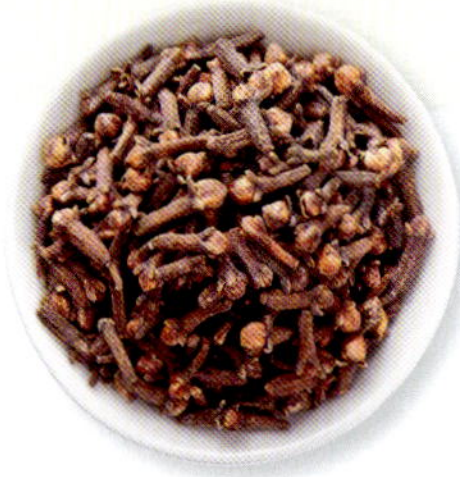

(Latin Name: *Caryophyllus aromaticus, Eugenia aromatica*)

The tangy essence is derived from the unopened buds of a fragrant evergreen native to the Moluccas and was sprinkled on handkerchiefs. During the plague years of the Middle Ages and again during the nineteenth century, essence of clove was used as a purifying agent. Later, scientists discovered that clove oil kills typhoid germs and destroys bacteria.

A popular folk remedy for toothache is to apply this mildly antiseptic oil directly to the gums until you can see the dentist. In fact, my own dentist sometimes uses it in fillings and crowns. Clove oil also helps get rid of athlete's foot and other fungal infections.

The warm and sweetly spicy taste of clove combines well with many foods, including meat, chicken, and apples. In potion-crafting, you can add cloves to spiced cider, warm milk drinks, liqueurs, broths, and curries.

Like other spices, cloves have acquired a reputation as an aphrodisiac. The buds also are alleged to help nurture friendships and bring comfort and solace to those suffering the loss of a loved one.

GINGER

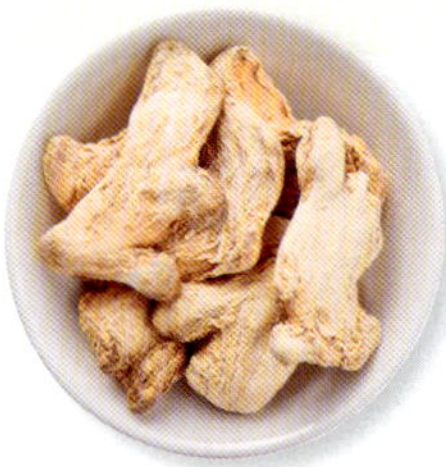

(Latin Name: *Zingiber officinale*)

Like most spices, ginger is a perennial tropical plant. The aromatic knobby rootstalks are the part used in cooking. Besides flavoring liquid potions such as sauces, ginger beer, and ginger wine, this versatile culinary spice adds zest to biscuits, breads, cakes, cookies, fish, fruit, meat, and pies. My favorite carbonated drink is homemade ginger lemonade.

I find that drinking a ginger infusion aids my digestion, banishes headaches, and quells motion sickness. This spice stimulates the digestion, so it can encourage weight loss. Ginger is also an expectorant used to alleviate congestion from coughs and colds.

In potion-crafting, some herbalists consider it a remedy for frigidity. This botanical also helps develop the intuitive faculties. Add it to potions when you want quick results.

MUSTARD

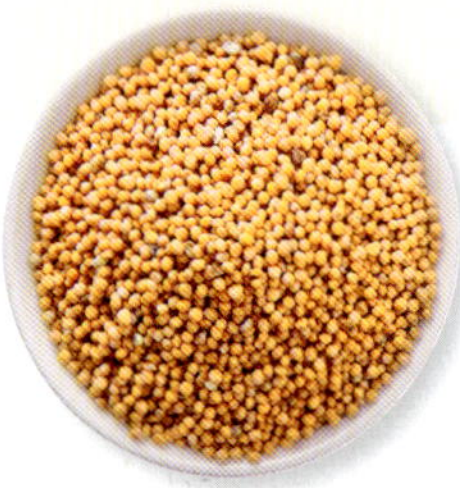

(Latin Name: *Brassica alba, Yellow Mustard; B. nigra, Black Mustard*)

Mustard plants are native to the wastelands of Egypt, Syria, and the Mediterranean. Several varieties also grow wild in the Western US. I've saved many a savory sauce by adding a touch of mustard.

The seed, which is the part most often used, is a carminative, diuretic, emetic, and stimulant. It sterilizes and deodorizes because it destroys bacteria. In days gone by, mustard plaster was a renowned home remedy for coughs and colds.

Mustard is associated with the planet Mars and the zodiac sign Aries. As such, it is an ingredient of potions to strengthen the mental and physical bodies.

NUTMEG

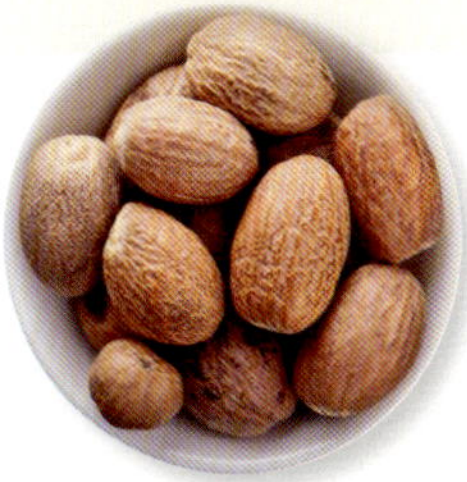

(Latin Name: *Myristica fragrans, Nux moschata*)

The kernel of this tropical fruit is a beloved culinary spice that adds warmth to milk-based potions. Nutmeg also stimulates the gastrointestinal tract. Used externally, it invigorates sore muscles and joints. The kernel is also slightly narcotic. In fact, nutmeg is poisonous in large doses and may cause miscarriage.

As a key ingredient of love potions, nutmeg was much favored by Napoleon and Josephine. Add it to brews to increase wealth, improve business, and win at the lottery. Here is a nutmeg potion to enjoy, especially at the winter holidays.

Serves 2

NUTMEG EGGNOG

Ingredients

- 1 egg
- 1 teaspoon organic sugar
- 1 cup fat-free milk
- ¼ teaspoon vanilla
- Nutmeg

Directions

Beat the egg until it becomes light and foamy. Add the sugar and beat again until the mixture is thick and lemon-colored. Gradually blend in milk and vanilla. Pour into a glass and sprinkle with ground nutmeg. Serve in 2 punch glasses. Yum!

Herbal Infusions

Herbal beverages have been brewed since primitive times, both as refreshments and remedies. Chinese medicine is based, in part, on prescribing strong herbal brews called decoctions. In general, strong-tasting concoctions rarely enter into culinary potion-crafting. Instead, we drink herbal infusions otherwise known as tisanes. An herbal infusion or tisane are traditional names for beverage infusions composed of single or blended botanicals that are not derived from the *Camellia sinensis* bush. They are brewed much like tea, and this is one reason many people refer to them as herbal teas.

Hundreds of botanicals exist from which enticing brews can be concocted. Depending on the specific botanical, infusions can be made from all parts of the plant including flower, seed, stem, root, and rhizome, with the leaf being the most ubiquitous ingredient. Combinations are truly endless and showcase how well Mother Nature has provided for humanity.

Because these brews provide small amounts of essential vitamins and minerals, many people drink them for their nutritional benefits. Just think of

Hercule Poirot, the brilliant but fussy Belgian detective of the Agatha Christie mysteries, who felt he could not possibly live without his daily tisane. Throughout this book, and especially in Appendix A, you will find references to the health benefits of many of these botanicals.

Although the action of herbal beverages is generally subtle and mild, infusions can produce the same effects on your body as dietary supplements. Therefore, I recommend you always tell your health professional about any botanicals you plan to drink as health potions. Your doctor will know if any of the herbs interfere with your prescribed medications or which could have a deleterious effect on a condition you may be suffering. Children and pregnant women should pay special attention to this advice, as some botanicals that are safe for the general population can harm their delicate constitutions.

How to Prepare an Herbal Infusion

The process for creating herbal infusions is similar to what you learned in Chapter 4 for brewing beverage teas. To make an herbal infusion, add 1 to 2 fresh chopped sprigs or ½ teaspoon dried flowers and leaves to 1 cup of cold water. Many herbalists recommend using fresh spring water or filtered water, but this is not necessary. Bring to a boil in a nonmetal container, then lower heat. Cover the container with a lid so the essential oils do not escape and simmer for 3–5 minutes. Transfer the liquid to a mug, straining away the herbs.

Boil and simmer for twice the amount of time if you are brewing from roots, barks, and seeds, as it takes a longer brewing time to release their essence.

Some tea masters shrink from the notion of boiling the water because they maintain that boiling scorches the delicate leaves and evaporates the essential oils. They recommend that if you must boil the water, you should wait for the water to cool for a couple of minutes before adding the herbs. I have not seen how this makes any difference in the quality of my infusions. However, I live at high altitude and water boils at a lower temperature here.

For a description of twelve terrific tisane herbs and their uses, see Appendix B on page 179.

Sara's Elementary Tisanes

Since in Chapter 1, I discussed the importance of the four elements of nature for potion-crafting, it seems appropriate to end this part of the book with tisane recipes for each element. By drinking these infusions, we become more mindful of the elements and incorporate some of their qualities and strengths into our bodies. We can also increase our odds of remaining healthy, wealthy, and wise, and live in harmony with the natural world around us for a long time to come. Such a deal!

Sara Martinelli, a certified tea master, herbalist, and restaurateur, has graciously offered to share her delicious Tisanes of the Four Elements ingredients. Amounts are given in bulk so that you'll only need to remake these recipes every month or so. Store what you don't use in an airtight container to keep the blends fresh. Remember to label your container.

Air Element TISANE

Ingredients

- ¼ cup lemon verbena
- ¼ cup peppermint
- ⅛ cup dandelion leaf
- ⅛ cup lemongrass
- 2 teaspoon aniseed
- 1 teaspoon lavender

Water Element TISANE

Ingredients

- ½ cup chamomile
- ¼ cup jasmine
- ¼ cup blackberry leaf
- ⅛ cup spearmint
- 1 tablespoon skullcap
- 1 tablespoon rose hips
- 1 teaspoon licorice root, cut
- 1 teaspoon lemon peel
- ½ teaspoon hibiscus

Fire Element TISANE

Ingredients

- ¼ cup Siberian ginseng
- ¼ cup peppermint
- ¼ cup hawthorn berries, slightly ground
- 1 tablespoon orange peel
- 1 tablespoon calendula petals
- 1 tablespoon cinnamon chips
- 1 tablespoon fennel
- ½ teaspoon nutmeg
- ½ teaspoon clove, ground

Earth Element TISANE

Ingredients

- ¼ cup alfalfa
- ¼ cup nettle leaf
- ⅛ cup oat straw
- 1 tablespoon mugwort

In the next part of this book you'll find scores of recipes for liquid potions to help you obtain everything from a marriage proposal to securing the perfect internship, jump-starting your creativity, and improving your health.

Part II

POTIONS FOR ALL OCCASIONS

In this section you'll find all kinds of potions from smoothies to enthuse you to snag the job of your dreams, to a night cap tisane that will guarantee a restful sleep, a mocha malt to help ace that important test, and a tea to facilitate communication between you and your pet, as well as wildlife. Not only do these drinks taste good, they're good for you!

Notice that several recipes include pinches of the herbs and spices I introduced in Chapter 6. I've tried to keep the number of different herbs to a minimum so you don't feel you must stock an apothecary in your kitchen. Many of these botanicals are ascribed multiple esoteric attributes anyway because our ancestors had more limited access to varieties of herbs than we do.

Some recipes call for juiced fruits and vegetables. Personally, I find juicing worthwhile. But you don't need to run out and buy a juicer if you don't already have one or don't have the time to juice every ingredient from scratch. Many fine juices of all sorts are readily available at most grocery stores, and there's no shame in taking a shortcut. If you decide to use commercially prepared juices, I recommend you buy organic brands with no sugar added.

I also advise you to stay away from juices packaged in plastic bottles stamped with PET or PETE (Polyethylene Terephthalate). *Consumer Reports* (December 1, 2011) has found that this kind of plastic can leak carcinogens such as arsenic, lead, antimony, and phthalates into the contents, especially into apple juice. I don't want to alarm you because this problem does not occur in all of these types of bottles and the levels that do exist are not necessarily dangerously high. If you or someone you know is especially sensitive to these substances, you may want to give these kinds of bottles a miss and go for glass containers.

One way to approach this section is to thumb through the chapters. Familiarize yourself with the different kinds of potions, their general ingredients, and the equipment you'll need. Each chapter stands alone and tells a little story. The recipes conform to the chapter's theme. Pick and choose recipes to try according to your intentions. In no time you'll be using the recipes simply as a guide and will enjoy experimenting on your own. This is why at the end of many of the recipes, I list alternative ingredients.

As you master the art of potion-crafting, you may want to turn to Part III. This compendium of scores of ingredients will add to your stockpot of potion knowledge.

Ready to immerse yourself in the delicious realm of love? Look to Chapter 7.

Chapter 7

SOMEDAY MY PRINCE (OR PRINCESS) WILL COME

Photograph by C. Nathan Pulley Photography

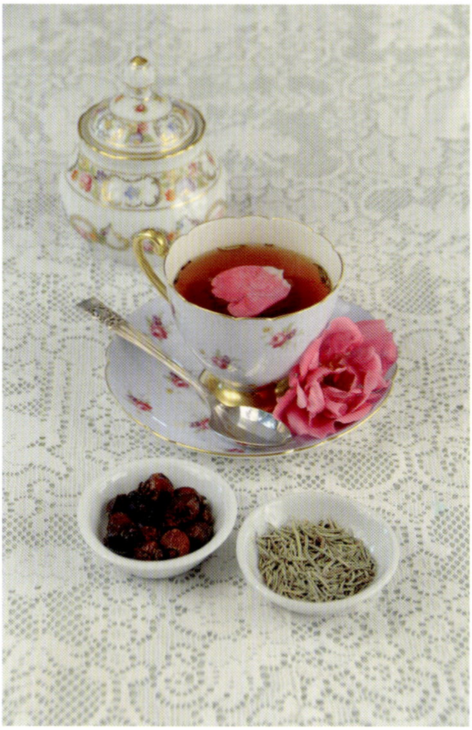

Come to Me Soul Mate Potion.

Potions for Amorous Relationships

The greatest thing you will ever learn is just to love and be loved in return.
–Eden Ahbez (1908–1995), Lyricist
From the song "Nature Boy"

Ask anyone on the street to relay what they know about potions, and the first types they'll probably mention are formulas to draw love. The concept of love extends far beyond simply attracting a mate, although this makes a good beginning. In this chapter you will find recipes centered on many facets of love.

Serves 1

Looking for Love TISANE

Starting with basics, let's suppose you have yet to meet Mr. or Ms. Right, and you're getting frustrated by the lack of response. Prepare yourself a cup of the following tea.

Ingredients

- 1 cup hot water
- ½ teaspoon rose hips, crushed
- ¼ teaspoon pink rose petals, whole (dried or fresh)
- ¼ teaspoon lovage, cut and sifted
- ¼ teaspoon vervain, cut and sifted

Directions

Make a beverage infusion from the ingredients and drink it hot before leaving home in the morning. Look forward to the special opportunities that the day may bring.

Serves 1

Come-to-Me SOUL MATE POTION

You've dated around, but that very special person–the one and only–has yet to put in an appearance. This updated version of a fifteenth-century attraction potion may help increase your odds.

Ingredients

- 1 cup hot water
- ½ teaspoon Orange Pekoe tea (or 1 Orange Pekoe teabag)
- ¼ teaspoon marjoram
- 1 rose petal, torn
- ¼ teaspoon honey
- ¼ teaspoon rose hips, crushed
- 2 drops almond essence

Directions

Drink before retiring to dream of your future mate. Note that both of the above recipes include rose hips, which are jam-packed with vitamin C. These infusions will keep you healthy and improve your skin tone so you will look your most appealing. (See photo at beginning of chapter.)

OTHER SOUL MATE BOTANICALS

Almond, Olive leaf, Yarrow, Olive, Jasmine flower

Serves 1

Unite E-mail LOVERS CIDER

Perhaps you're the sort of person, who when it comes to attracting a mate, is weary of the social scene. You wish you could meet someone from the comfort and security of your computer or mobile device. Here's an old formula that adapts well to the twenty-first century cyber world.

Ingredients

- 1 cup apple cider
- 1 teaspoon dried honeysuckle flower (or substitute whole cloves, crushed)
- Licorice stick

Directions

Prepare a cup of hot apple cider and add 1 teaspoon of dried honeysuckle flowers. If you can't find dried honeysuckle flowers, substitute a couple of crushed whole cloves. Stir the cider with a licorice stick, then turn on your computer or mobile device. Stir and sip your drink while chatting online.

OTHER BOTANICALS TO FACILITATE ANY TYPE OF COMMUNICATION

Lemon balm Persimmon Rosemary

Serves 1

Conquer My Jealous Heart INFUSION

If you're like me, initially you may have some trouble viewing your rival in the beatifically forgiving way as described in the last recipe. If you are still tortured by pangs of jealousy, here's a potion to help cleanse away those negative emotions.

Ingredients

- 1 cup hot water
- 1 peppermint teabag
- 3 coriander seeds, crushed

Directions

Add the coriander to the hot water with the teabag and steep for 3 to 5 minutes. Drink this herbal tisane whenever you find yourself overcome by spasms of jealousy or envy.

Eating olives (green ones, of course, for they symbolize the green-eyed monster) is also reputed to soothe an aching heart.

Serves 1 (with possible leftovers)

SPECIAL DATE JUICE

Photograph by C. Nathan Pulley Photography

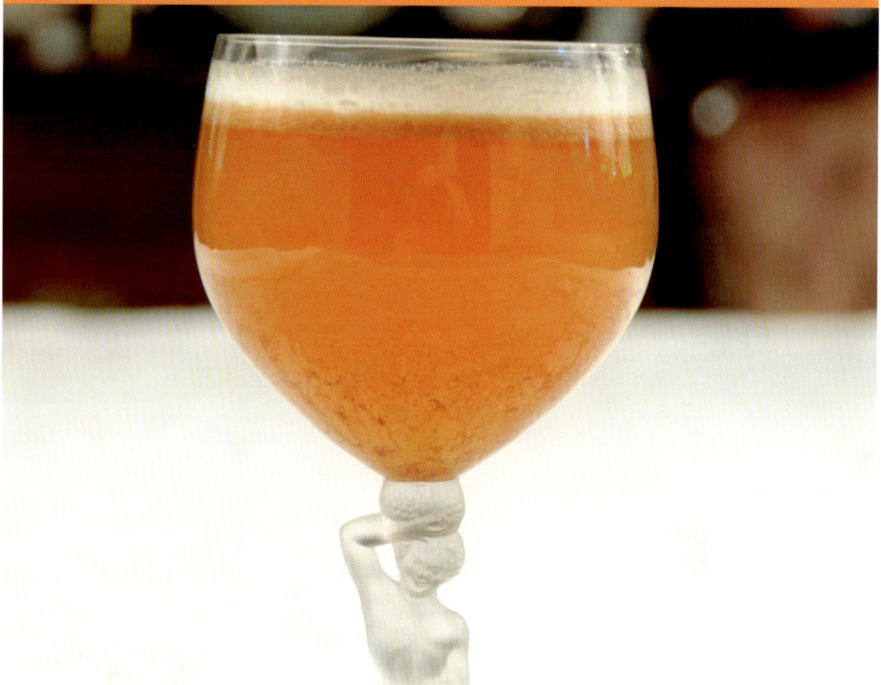

Hurray! You've met an intriguing candidate and are about to sally forth on a first date. To help make the occasion memorable, enjoy the following!

Ingredients

- 1 cup white grape juice, chilled
- ½ cup pear juice
- ¼ cup coconut water
- ½ teaspoon vanilla extract
- ¼ teaspoon ginseng extract (or 1 envelope instant ginseng tea dissolved in ¼ cup boiling water and cooled)
- ¼ teaspoon cinnamon
- 1 egg white, optional
- 3 ice cubes
- Honeydew slices for garnish
- Bing cherries (pitted) for garnish

Directions

Liquify the ingredients in a blender until frothy and pour into a tall glass with a garnish of honeydew slices and bing cherries (pitted) on a skewer. You don't have to drink this potion all at once. Store leftovers in the fridge.

OTHER "SPECIAL DATE" FRUITS

Blueberry

Fig

Passion fruit
(one of my favorites)

Pineapple
(also reputed to help bring back a straying lover)

Raspberry

Serves 2

Passion's Plaything

PASSION FRUIT SAUCE

The dinner-and-movie date was awesome, and ever since you've enjoyed each other's company often. Now it's time to get a tad more intimate. To that end, you've invited your special someone for a home-cooked meal. To top off the dinner and help make things happen, I recommend the following ice cream sauce.

Ingredients

- 4 ripe passion fruits
- Honey, stevia (or sugar) to taste
- 2 scoops (or more) vanilla ice cream

Directions

Halve the fruits, scoop out the pulp, and put through a sieve to remove the seeds. Cook with the sweetener over a low fire until the mixture thickens slightly and you have a fresh-tasting sauce.

If this seems like too much trouble, buy a bottle of passion fruit juice and enough cornstarch to thicken into a sauce when you heat it over a low fire.

Serve in wineglasses over vanilla ice cream, and if possible, sit together in front of a cozy fire. Now watch the sparks fly and feel the sizzle!

OTHER BOTANICALS TO INCREASE PASSION

Asparagus
Beet
Cardamom
Cinnamon
Cherry
Clove
Coriander
Cubeb berry
Damiana
Dill seeds
Elecampane
Ginger (also alleged to cure frigidity)
Red grape (or red wine)
Kava-kava
Ketchup
Lettuce
Lotus root
Passion flower
Raspberry
Rose
Tomato

Serves 1

Eliminate a Rival (in a Kind Way) SMOOTHIE

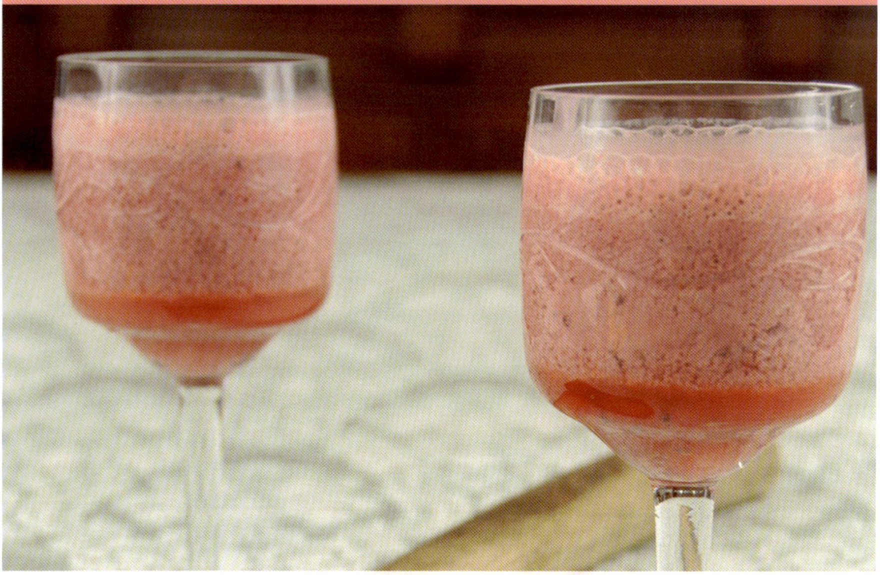

Photograph by C. Nathan Pulley Photography

Sparks have flown, but to your chagrin you find that your lover's former flame has been prowling around. How to rid yourself of the dreaded rival without incurring a terrible karmic debt? The following suggestion may be difficult to follow, but I promise the result will be worthwhile. As you prepare this juice, focus on *positive thoughts* about your nemesis. Make a mental list of the person's better qualities. None of those negative, vengeful sentiments, thank you! They'll only hurt you in the end. We all have our good points, even our enemies. So visualize this person attaining his or her full potential, only in another location, field of endeavor, and most importantly, with another more suitable partner.

Ingredients

- 1 cup orange juice
- ½ cup cranberry juice
- ½ cup blackberries
- ½ cup ice
- 1 cup low fat vanilla or fat-free Greek yogurt
- 1-2 tablespoons honey

Directions

Place the juices, blackberries, and ice in a blender and mix on low speed until blended. Add the yogurt and honey; continue mixing, gradually increasing the speed until the mixture is smooth. Pour the blend into glasses and garnish with a slice of orange.

Here comes the hard part. Offer a glass to your rival. As you share the potion, express your desire to bury the hatchet. Have faith that the person will soon find another love interest, and you will come out the winner.

Toast to the Bride and Groom

Congratulations! You've made it to the altar. To get your marriage off to a super start, at the reception make sure you have plenty of cherry juice on hand (or Kirsch liqueur, an alcoholic beverage based on cherries). Have a good friend or relative offer the toast. Kir Champagne also works well. (See the recipe in Chapter 17.)

Other traditional wedding botanicals, some of which, besides being potion ingredients, can be tucked into the bride's bouquet:

- Linden
- Orange blossom
- Vervain,
- Onion

Personally, I wouldn't include this last ingredient in the bouquet. If you're disposed to eating onions on your wedding night, make sure both you and your partner sample them.

Serves 2

Make up After a Quarrel COOLER

Uh-oh! Married life, though mostly blissful, has its occasional ups-and-downs. You've suffered through your first tiff. It wasn't serious and now you're making up. Cool your tempers and celebrate your renewed ardor with this drink.

Ingredients

- 2 cups boiling water
- 2 black teabags (any variety)
- 1 almond teabag (Lipton used to make almond tea, but I haven't seen it lately. If you can't find it, substitute ¼ teaspoon almond extract)
- ½ pint orange sherbet
- ½ banana

Directions

Prepare an infusion from 2 cups of boiling water, and the black and almond teabags. Remove the bags and set aside. If you garden, use the spent bags later as fertilizer. Chill tea for 4 hours. To serve, put the tea through a blender with the sherbet, banana, and almond extract, if you're using it. Pour into tall glasses. This cooler also is alleged to turn a friend into a lover.

OTHER BOTANICALS TO HELP PATCH OLD EMOTIONAL WOUNDS

Caraway
Pear
Rue
Spikenard
Violet

Serves 2

Amiable Parting of the Ways HERBAL INFUSION

Perhaps you have not exactly followed the path to true love and happiness as outlined above. To quote the Bible, "To everything there is a season." Sometimes it is better to accept a parting of the ways than to keep making each other miserable. To show you bear no ill will, offer your "ex" a final cup of tea, and reminisce over the good times. Prepare a beverage infusion in 2 cups of hot water.

Ingredients

- 1 teaspoon peppermint, fresh, chopped (½ teaspoon if dried)
- 1 teaspoon lemon balm, fresh, chopped (½ teaspoon if dried)
- (Organic or demerara sugar, to taste)

Directions

To remind you of the fond memories, add organic or demerara sugar to taste, if desired. Pour into mugs and serve. Here's to the good times!

Due to limited space, the above recipes do not address every imaginable kind of amorous relationship. For ideas to follow up on your own, here is a list of other ingredients. These botanicals have been popular over the ages to attract love, foster affection and friendship, and create harmonious relationships:

Angelica	Cabbage	Cucumber	Leek	Solomon's seal
Anise	Carrot	Damiana	Maidenhair	Spikenard
Apricot	Celery	Elecampane	Mushroom	Sugar
Artichoke	Chocolate	Juniper	Papaya	Tarragon
Basil	Cinquefoil	Kava-kava	Parsley	Thyme

If you've been successful meeting your true love, you're going to want some extra cash for special dates, clothes, and sundries, not to mention a good, steady job. The next chapter on money and prosperity may hold special interest for you.

Chapter 8

I NEED MONEY, HONEY! POTIONS FOR WEALTH AND PROSPERITY

> Money.
> You don't know where it's been/
> but you put it where your mouth is/and it talks.
> –Dana Gioia (b. 1950)
> Poet, critic, translator

Next to love, money and prosperity probably rank at the top of most people's wish lists, especially in these days of economic hard times. If you're hankering after wealth and want to concoct a potion to speed you to your goal, permit me to share a few pearls of wisdom based on my experiences.

First, I recommend you count the blessings you already possess. When you add up everything you have to your credit, the debit side probably won't look so bad. Next, quit obsessing over scarcity, poverty, and bad luck. Think rich and powerful! And remember to practice charity every day of your life, for what goes around, comes around.

Also, I suggest you be mindful of the spiritual side of prosperity. Material manifestations are simply the results of what has already occurred on the spiritual plane.

You can do a lot of practical things to draw prosperity to your life. Establish goals and strive to bring them to fruition. You'll notice that the harder you work, the luckier you'll get. This is no coincidence. Nobody is going to hand you treasures on a silver platter.

As we get down to the nitty-gritty of potion-crafting for wealth acquisition, I am going to sound like a worried parent and order you to eat (or in this case, drink) your greens. Green is the color of money, fecundity, and prosperity. The more green foods you infuse into your body such as peas, lettuce, broccoli, and avocados, the more wealth you will attract. And did I mention that green foods are really good for you?

When rustling up a prosperity potion, I suggest you use your five senses that I talked about in Chapter 1:

1. Visualize wealth;
2. Evoke the scent of crisp bills in your hands;
3. Hear with your mind's ear the coins clinking merrily in your pocket;
4. Savor the taste, and
5. Texture of your potion as you drink, for this is the rich, velvety flavor of abundance.

Bearing all of this in mind, let's move on to some recipes to draw wealth and prosperity for specific situations.

Serves 1

Dollars and Cents TEA

Ingredients

- 1 cup hot water
- ¼ teaspoon chamomile flowers, dried
- ¼ teaspoon peppermint leaves, dried
- Pinch of basil
- 1 green teabag

Directions

For general prosperity, infuse ¼ teaspoon of dried chamomile flowers, ¼ teaspoon of dried peppermint leaves, and a pinch of basil, along with 1 green teabag in a cupful of hot water. Drink this infusion first thing each morning until your situation improves.

If you want to add an extra kick to your good luck at lotto or other games of chance, wash your hands in the tea (cool it first!) before leaving home to play cards (or bingo!) or to purchase lottery tickets. This is such an easy potion to concoct and so tasty, that you might want to make up a large jar of it so you can scoop out 1 teaspoonful at a time whenever you want it.

Makes several servings

Sun Shine on Me Today DAY TEA

Like the Sun dawning on a brand-new day, this refreshing tea opens your mind and intuition to new opportunities as they present themselves.

Ingredients

- 2 teaspoons Lady Grey Green tea (any brand, but choose the kind flavored with Seville oranges rather than the kind flavored with lavender)
- ½ teaspoon lemon balm leaves (fresh or ¼ teaspoon dried)
- ½ teaspoon wheatgrass
- ¼ teaspoon ginseng powder
- ¼ teaspoon guaraná seeds, crushed
- ⅛ teaspoon chia seed, crushed
- Pinch of safflower (or saffron, although saffron is expensive)
- Squirt of fresh lemon

Directions

Mix together all of the ingredients except the lemon, and store in an airtight spice jar. Depending on how strong you take your tea, this recipe will render several cups. I, for one, only use ½ teaspoon per cup of hot water. Add a squirt or two of lemon to each serving.

Serves 1

CARROT JUICE
Potion

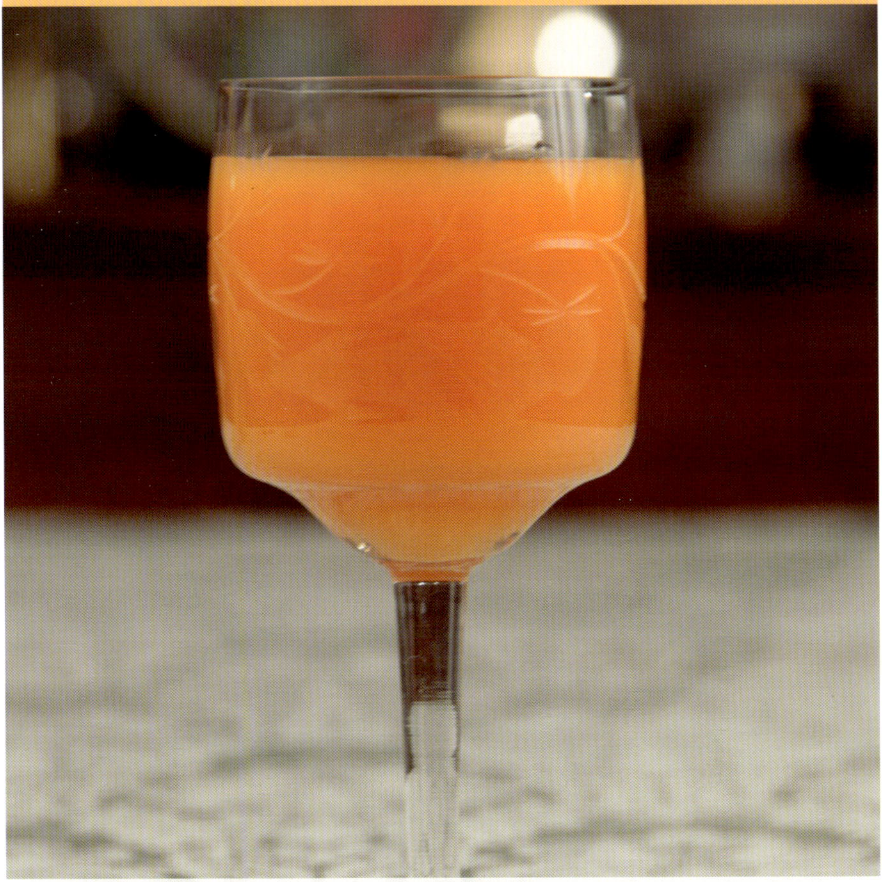

Photograph by C. Nathan Pulley Photography

One of the simplest and healthiest ways to draw prosperity throughout the day is to drink a glass of carrot juice for breakfast.

Ingredients

- 1 glass carrot juice, organic or self-juiced
- Pinch or two of ginger, ground or freshly grated

Directions

Either juice it yourself or buy organic juice at the grocery. To infuse your efforts with spice, add a pinch or two of ground or freshly grated ginger. Contemplate the worry-free, affluent life you want to live. While sipping, repeat silently the following affirmation:

Serves 4

Luck o' the Irish
CHOCO-MINT SHAKE

Poor Mr. Jones! So you don't end up feeling as he does, here's a potion purported to guide you to pick lucky lotto numbers. Mind you, I make no promises, but please do remember me when you hit the jackpot!

Ingredients

- 1 pint chocolate frozen yogurt
- ½ cup nonfat milk
- 1 teaspoon vanilla extract
- ¼ teaspoon nutmeg, ground
- 6 drops mint extract (If you prefer alcohol in your shake, substitute 2 tablespoons of crème de menthe)
- Fresh peppermint garnish, if desired

Directions

Place the ingredients in a blender; cover, and blend well. Serve immediately in tall glasses. Decorate with sprigs of fresh peppermint leaves if desired.

Serves 2

Choose High Performance
STOCKS JUICE

Cherries, the main ingredient in this recipe are alleged to draw money and prosperity. The spices and coffee are thought to hone the perceptions.

Ingredients

- 1 cup pitted sweet cherries*
- Peppermint sprigs, for garnish
- Blend in:
- 1 tablespoon turbinado sugar
- ½ teaspoon instant coffee
- ½ teaspoon cinnamon powder
- ¼ teaspoon allspice powder

Directions

Pour into tall glasses, and garnish with peppermint sprigs.

*If you have a juicer, juice 1 cupful of pitted sweet cherries and add ¼ cup of water. If you don't own a juicer or cherries are out of season, substitute 2 cups of organic cherry juice. I prefer tart organic cherry juice, but if you use it, you may want to add more sweetener.

OTHER BOTANICALS ALLEGED TO DRAW GENERAL PROSPERITY AND WELL-BEING AND IMPROVE YOUR ECONOMIC CONDITIONS

Almond
Anise
Basil
Bay
Cardamom
Cinquefoil
Currant
Dandelion (leaf and root)
Ginseng
Honey
Mango
Papaya
Peas
Pomegranate
Solomon's seal

Serves 1

Count Your Blessings TEA

At the beginning of this chapter, I talked about counting the blessings you already have before going in search of more wealth.

The following recipe will help you remember the good things in life you already possess. As with most of the teas in these chapters that include several botanicals, you can make up more of this recipe than you need for 1 cup of tea. Store the rest in an airtight spice jar for future use.

Ingredients

- 1 tablespoon jasmine green tea
- 2 teaspoons lemon balm, dried and crushed
- 1 teaspoon angelica root, cut and sifted
- ¼ teaspoon cardamom powder

Directions

Mix the ingredients well, and use ½ teaspoon per cup of hot water.

Serves 1

Charity Begins at Home JUICE

As you take pleasure in your new-found prosperity, I remind you to also enjoy giving to those who are less fortunate. To encourage yourself to remember this, try the following juice.

Ingredients

- ⅔ cup grape juice
- ⅓ cup pear juice
- Pinch allspice (for compassion)
- Pinch spearmint (for transformation from poverty to wealth for others)

Directions

Pour into a glass, stir well, and drink.

BOTANICALS WITH SIMILAR PROPERTIES

Carnation	Motherwort	Peas*
Lady's mantle	Olive	
Marjoram	Yam	

* Speaking of peas, for a Prosperous New Year Pea Soup recipe, see Chapter 17.

Now that you're fortified with a positive, prosperous outlook, are you ready to tackle those knotty issues centered on career and goals? If so, read on.

Chapter 9

THE SKY'S THE LIMIT

Potions for Career and Goals

Maybe you're not a self-starter like Mr. Jordan; most of us need a nudge from time to time. Perhaps at the moment, your life is in flux and you're pinging from job to job. We all endure frustrating periods developing our careers. I know because I've done everything from housecleaning to babysitting, data entry, translation, interpretation, mail order, retail, aromatherapy, university teaching, intercultural training, assessment, candle-making, and tea-blending. Finally, I hit on my ideal career as a writer. Throughout each phase, I have had to learn to focus and refocus my aspirations.

> I've missed more than 9,000 shots in my career. I've lost almost 300 games. 26 times, I've been trusted to take the game winning shot and missed. I've failed over and over and over again in my life. And that is why I succeed.
> –Michael Jordan (b. 1962)
> NBA star

Which is the best way to identify and achieve your goals? In the first place, it won't help to fret over what you want or how you're going to get it. Once you've decided on an objective and put in the hard work to prepare to attain it, don't waste any more mental and emotional energy. Have faith in the universe. Out there time is not linear, so don't concern yourself with the sequence of events. The best recompense is happiness and a sense of personal fulfillment. This should be your ultimate aim.

The following juice potion will help you concentrate on your long-term goals. I also recommend protein-rich food or supplements to smooth the progress toward focusing your brain. Try adding protein powders to your favorite juices and smoothies, even if they are not included in many of these recipes. While you're whipping up this potion, contemplate this quote from Hannibal, the second-century BCE conqueror, *"We will either find a way or make one."*

Serves 1

Secure a Fascinating Internship VITAMINAS

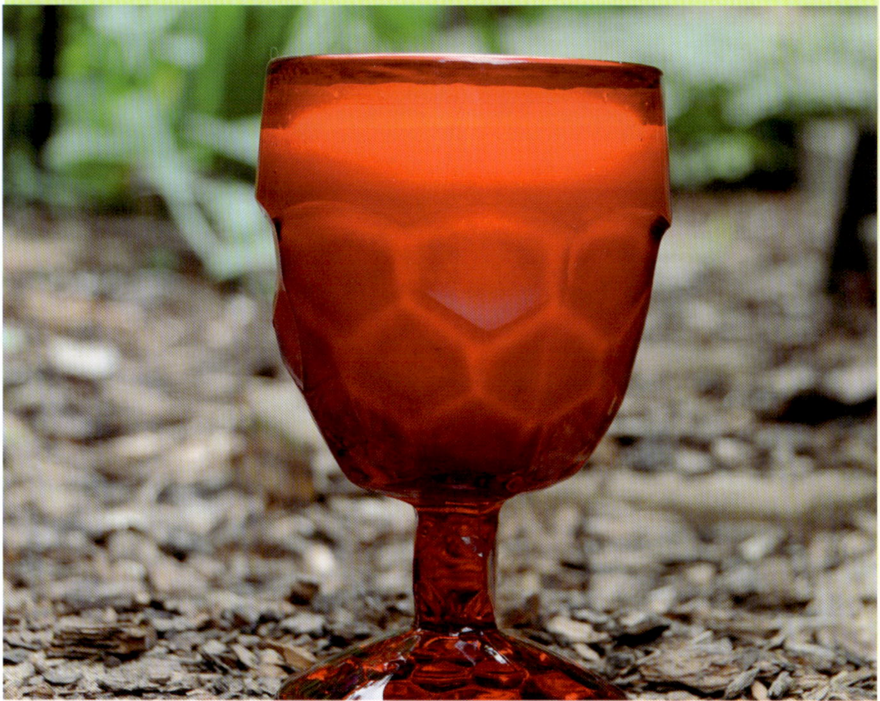

Photograph by C. Nathan Pulley Photography

Before you embark on the interview circuit, you may feel the need to acquire additional skills and experience. Perhaps you're starting out in your career, coming back on the market after a long absence, or simply desire a change of scene. Why not get the necessary training to vault up the ladder by serving as an intern? To put you in the proper frame of mind to begin your search for the right internship, try this popular Brazilian *Vitaminas* recipe. Its main ingredient is banana, a wish-fulfillment fruit. The cinnamon is believed to produce swift action.

Ingredients

- 1 cup whole milk
- 1 small banana, peeled and chopped
- ½ cup old-fashioned oats
- 2 tablespoons vanilla-flavored protein powder (optional)
- ½ teaspoon cinnamon
- 3–4 ice cubes

Directions

Place all of the ingredients in a blender, cover, and mix well. Pour the potion into a glass. Drink it down, hit the road, and conquer your goal.

Serves 2 or more

Open My Paths JUICE

Photograph by C. Nathan Pulley Photography

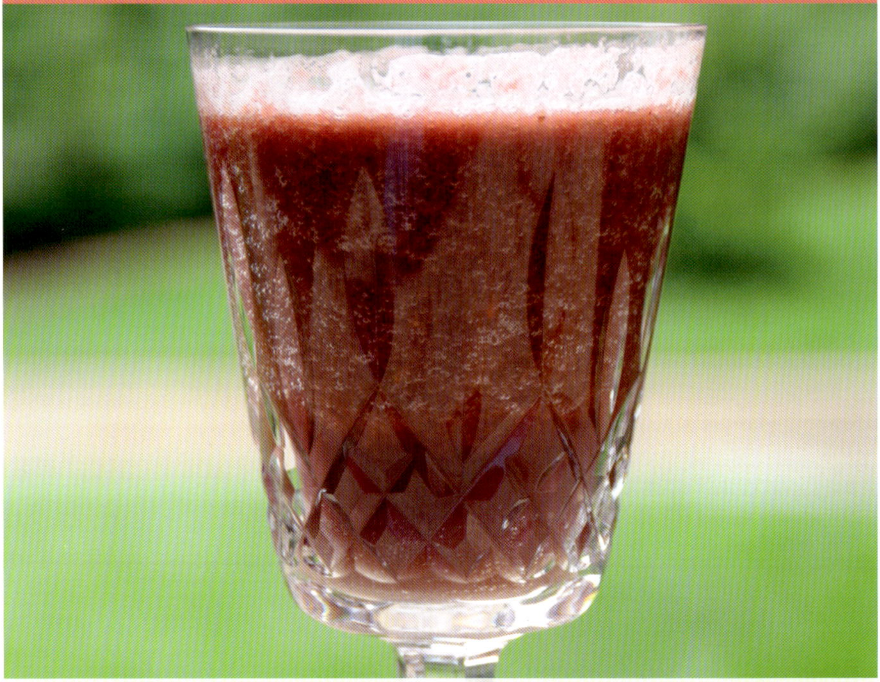

This potion relies on blackberries to open windows of opportunity and helps you choose the wise path. Cantaloupe enhances your creativity to make the most of your choice, and ginseng instills you with energy to follow through.

Ingredients

- 1 cup blackberries
- 1 cup cantaloupe, scooped from the rind, cubed
- 1 apple, peeled, cored, and cut into eighths
- 1 packet instant ginseng tea dissolved in ¼ cup water
- Sweetener of your choice, to taste
- Sprig lavender, for garnish if desired

Directions

If you can't find the instant variety of the ginseng tea, make a decoction from a ginseng tea bag. That is to say, place the bag in 1 cup of boiling water and keep boiling until you reduce the liquid to ¼ cup. Refrigerate for 1 hour before adding to the juice.

Place the fruit in your juicer, alternating blackberries, cantaloupe, and apples; process until juiced. Add the ginseng tea and blend again. If you want to drink the juice very cold, throw in a few cubes of ice, or use frozen blackberries. If the fruit is not sweet enough, sweeten to taste. Pour the juice into glasses. Garnish with blackberries or strawberries, and a sprig of lavender, if desired. The ginseng in this juice also stands for renewal.

OTHER USEFUL BOTANICALS TO OPEN YOUR PATHS:

Leeks (a mild onion-like vegetable popular in the British Isles that stands for clear-headedness)
Celery (for grounding)

Serves approximately 2-4

WHITE GRAPE
Determination Potion

Assuming you have identified your goal, it's time to follow through with increased determination. Here's a potion:

Ingredients

- 1 pint white grape juice (or white wine, if you prefer an alcoholic beverage)
- 1 teaspoon juniper berries, crushed

Directions

Pour the juice into a bottle. Add the crushed juniper berries to the juice and refrigerate. Shake the bottle twice daily, remembering to replace it in the refrigerator. After one week, strain away the berries. Drink a small juice glassful of the liquid every morning. This potion is also alleged to enhance virility.

If this potion doesn't appeal, prepare a cup of Gunpowder green tea and add ¼ teaspoon of any of the following ingredients: chamomile, dill weed, 2 crushed allspice berries. Serves 1.

Serves 2

Sweeten a Cranky
DISPOSITION JUICE

At last you've netted the perfect job. Only trouble is, one of your coworkers acts like an overwrought porcupine in a field of cactus. Maybe this person hated to see your predecessor go, or resents that you got the job they coveted. Or this associate may be suffering personal problems and is taking them out on colleagues. To cast balm over the troubled waters, create the following potion.

Ingredients

- 2 carrots (or bottled fresh carrot juice)
- 1 small handful of strawberries, fresh or frozen
- Honey, to taste, if needed
- Ice
- Sprig of lemon, violet flowers, or bing cherries, if desired

Directions

If juicing the carrots from scratch, add enough water to make a liquid. Carrot juice is sweet, but if you have a really cantankerous individual to placate, sweeten the juice even more with honey. Blend until frothy. Serve over ice in tall glasses, and garnish with a sprig of lemon balm, a couple of violet flowers, or big, fat bing cherries.

Serves 2

Find Your Dream Job SMOOTHIE

If you've ever been thrown on the mercy of the fickle job market, I'm sure I'm not telling you anything new when I say that applying for employment can be a stressful, frustrating experience. To facilitate your search, I suggest you first take time to gather your thoughts and visualize your ideal job. Imagine yourself thriving in the consummate working environment, feeling productive, creative, and content. When you can picture this in your mind's eye so perfectly that it seems almost real, it's time to back off and relax with the following smoothie potion. It will help calm your emotions, direct your attention, and enable you to highlight your many excellent qualities and skills without becoming too pushy when you head out on the interview circuit.

Ingredients

- 2 ripe persimmons, with rind peeled away, cut into wedges
- 2 tablespoons brown sugar
- 1 teaspoon fresh lemon balm, chopped (If you can't find fresh lemon balm, substitute freshly squeezed lemon juice.)*
- 1 cup frozen raspberries
- 2 cups non-fat frozen vanilla yogurt

Directions

Blend the first 4 ingredients to a slushy consistency. Add the frozen yogurt and blend, slowly increasing the speed until the mixture is smooth. Fill a tall glass and garnish with fresh raspberries and blueberries on a skewer or toothpick. Enjoy! You will have plenty left over for a relaxing reward when you return from your triumphant interview because this recipe serves 2.

* Lemon and lemon balm are both held to improve communication skills and produce quick action.

Serves 4

CUP OF CHEER with Coworkers

To facilitate harmonious relationships at work, assemble this potion, if possible, in the company kitchen blender. If they don't supply a blender, bring one from home. If more than four colleagues are in your group, you will need to multiply the ingredients accordingly.

Ingredients

- 2 cups cherries, stemmed and seeded
- 2 cups fat-free vanilla yogurt
- 1 cup white grape juice
- ½ cup sparkling water
- 2 tablespoons honey
- 1 teaspoon lime juice, freshly squeezed
- ½ teaspoon vanilla extract
- 1 teaspoon bee pollen

Directions

Blend the ingredients until smooth and pour into glasses (Styrofoam cups will do in a pinch). Cheers!

Serves 4

Leader of the Pack
BROCCOLI-GOUDA SOUP

Feel it's time to assert your authority over your team? Get them together for lunch and offer the following soup. If it is inconvenient or impossible to cook in the company kitchen, prepare the soup at home and reheat it at work.

Ingredients

- 1 bunch fresh broccoli, chopped
- 2 cups water
- 1 cup whole milk
- 1½ cups Gouda cheese, grated
- ½ teaspoon garlic (or more, if everyone likes the garlicky taste)
- ¼ teaspoon paprika
- ¼ teaspoon nutmeg
- Salt and pepper to taste

Directions

In a medium saucepan, bring to a boil the broccoli and water. Reduce the heat to medium, cover the saucepan, and cook for 15–20 minutes or until the broccoli is tender. Stir in the milk, cheese, garlic, paprika, nutmeg, salt, and pepper, until the cheese has melted. Cool mixture and process in a blender until smooth. Re-heat thoroughly. Pour into bowls and garnish with parsley or more grated cheese, if desired.

After my husband, who is not particularly fond of broccoli, read this recipe, he quipped that you will have proven your leadership ability if you get your group to actually drink this soup. I happen to think the recipe is delicious. After you try the recipe, blog me at www.carolinedowbooks.com and weigh in with your opinion.

Serves 2

Techno-Perfect
SMOOTHIE

If you're having trouble understanding the ins-and-outs of the Internet, computers, mobile devices, iPads, and other apparatus of today's fast paced, tech-savvy world, and you're not counting calories, this delicious smoothie may be the very thing to help keep you abreast of innovations and help you secure that coveted job.

Ingredients

- 1 cup canned figs, drained (Save the juice/ syrup for another potion.)
- 2 cups sweet cream or cinnamon ice cream

Directions

Blend until smooth. Pour into a glass and feed your brain (and tummy). Refrigerate leftovers.

As you scale great heights in your career—which I sincerely hope you will—remember this quote from Marilyn Monroe: *"A career is wonderful, but you can't curl up with it on a cold night."*

Chapter 10

"MIRROR, MIRROR, ON THE WALL"

Potions for Beauty and Self-Improvement

Beauty is not caused. It is.
–Emily Dickinson (1830–1886), American poet

After love and money, it seems more potions for beauty and self-improvement have come down to us over the ages than for any other intention. The following recipes may not transform you into an Angelina or a Brad, but they may help you think about how to put your best foot forward in the world.

Serves 1

MAYA APRICOT-AVOCADO Beauty Potion

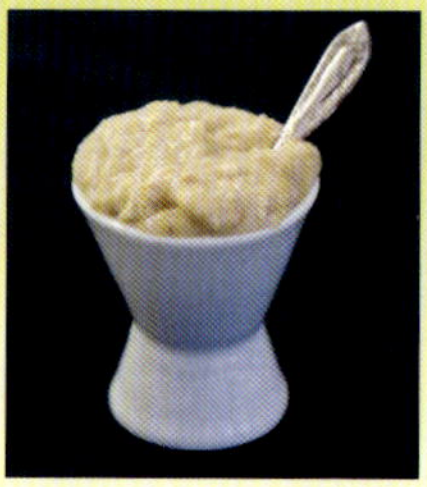

This ancient Maya inner-outer beauty formula calls for a blend of the following:

Ingredients

- ½ avocado, peeled and pitted
- 1 fresh apricot, pitted and quartered
- ½ cup water
- 1 tablespoon wheat germ
- 2–3 ice cubes
- Honey to taste

Directions

Pop everything in a blender, cover, and mix well. Pour into a glass and enjoy. Avocados nurture your body with plenty of potassium, apricots supply iron and copper, and wheat germ adds a shot of B vitamins.

If you leave out the ice cubes, this potion also makes an excellent facial masque. For a really moist masque, substitute olive oil for the water. Leave it on for 15-20 minutes before rinsing with cool water.

Serves 2

The Very Thing PINEAPPLE SMOOTHIE

Being well dressed elevates mood, brightens the outlook, and makes a person feel more confident. Let's say you want to find just the right item to wear to that key job interview from the last chapter or even for that special date from Chapter 7, an upcoming wedding, or class reunion. But you don't have time to browse the stores all day long or through the night online. Instead, take a few minutes to prepare and drink this smoothie before leaving on your shopping excursion or going to your browser, and perhaps the perfect ensemble will pop up before your eyes like magic. As an added benefit, this drink will fortify you physically for that marathon trek to the mall.

Ingredients

- ½ cup pineapple, cubed, fresh or canned
- ½ cup coconut water
- 2 tablespoons protein powder, vanilla-flavored
- 1 tablespoon black cherry syrup (available at most natural groceries—I order mine online from a reputable company)
- ¼ teaspoon almond extract
- ¼ teaspoon cinnamon
- 2 cups coconut frozen yogurt or ice cream

Directions

Place the first 4 ingredients in a blender and mix. Add the frozen yogurt or ice cream, and blend until smooth. Pour into a tall glass and enjoy. You might want to store one portion in the fridge to revive you on your triumphant return.

Serves 1

Mr./Ms. POPULARITY JUICE

When others enjoy your company, you bask in their approbation and become more beautiful from the inside-out. Being kind, courteous, and respectful goes a long way toward attracting others to your sparkling personality. If your personal appeal meter could use a boost, here's another apricot-based potion. According to folklore, this multi-talented fruit can coax your inner light to act as a beacon to draw new friends.

Ingredients

- ¼ cup apricot nectar
- ¼ cup skim milk
- 1 cup apricots, pitted and diced
- 1 tablespoon honey
- 2 pinches powdered cloves (to nurture friendship)
- 3 drops rosemary essence (If you can't find the essential oil, add 3 rosemary needles, chopped into bits.)

Directions

Blend all of the ingredients, pour into a tall glass, and serve over ice. Not only will you be popular, the rosemary will ensure that your breath is also sweet.

Serves 1

APRÈS
Sun and Ski Skin Toner

Prunes may be good for you to eat, but you don't want to end up looking like one from overexposure to sun. I probably don't need to remind you always to wear sunblock and take care not to par broil the largest organ of your body in those searing rays, especially at the beginning of the season. After a long day of fun in the sun at the beach, skiing, or gardening, the following recipe will help restore your parched epidermis to its natural healthy glow. It calls for aloe vera juice, which can taste quite bitter or not, depending on the brand. If you can't find a mild and tasty brand, you can offset the bitterness by adding honey. You can also increase the amount of strawberry juice, or simply substitute water. If you prefer, substitute for the aloe vera a combination of aloe vera juice and coconut water, available commercially.

Ingredients

- 1 cup aloe vera juice (or water, or combination of aloe vera and coconut water)
- ¼ cup strawberry juice
- 1 tablespoon rose hips, crushed
- 1-600 mg vitamin E capsule
- 1-500 mcg evening oil of primrose capsule

Directions

Place the first 2 ingredients in a blender. Squeeze out the contents of the 2 capsules, and liquefy. Pour into a glass and drink.

Serves 2

TRANQUILITY JUICE

Maybe you've tried the last formula, but still feel a bit nervy and unsettled. To calm your emotions and gain peace of mind, drink a glassful of the following juice.

Ingredients

- 2 apples, peeled, cored, and cut into eighths
- 1 pear, peeled, seeded and halved

Directions

Again, if you don't want to use a juicer, you can buy the organic juices. Alternate adding apples and pears to the juicer, and process until juiced. Add ¼ cup of sparkling water and blend. Garnish with fresh hibiscus flowers or cranberries, if available. Store leftovers in the fridge.

OTHER FOODS WITH PURPORTED TRANQUILIZING EFFECTS:

Cauliflower
Honey
Lettuce
Lime
Olive
Passion fruit
Potato

Herbs that produce similar effects:
Betony
Chamomile
Life everlasting (to gain peace mind)
Lady's mantle (for self-control)
Lavender (for balancing)
Poppy
Valerian

See Chapter 11 for more ideas.

Serves 1

CROSS-PATCH PREVENTION TEA

Photograph by C. Nathan Pulley Photography

The expression "ugly mood" wasn't coined for no good reason. When people feel out of sorts, their faces reflect inner turmoil. Crow's feet break out around the corners of the eyes, the eyebrows knit to create vertical lines between the eyes, and the corners of the mouth droop in a frown. If you can improve your mood on the inside, your facial expression, posture, and entire being will be transformed. Whenever you feel a hissy fit coming on, or find you're getting bossy or petty, quaff this tea. You can also sprinkle it (cooled) on your temples and at the back of your neck to help release tension. This potion is designed to help elicit the compassionate side of your nature and calm your nerves. Infuse it in 1 cup of hot water.

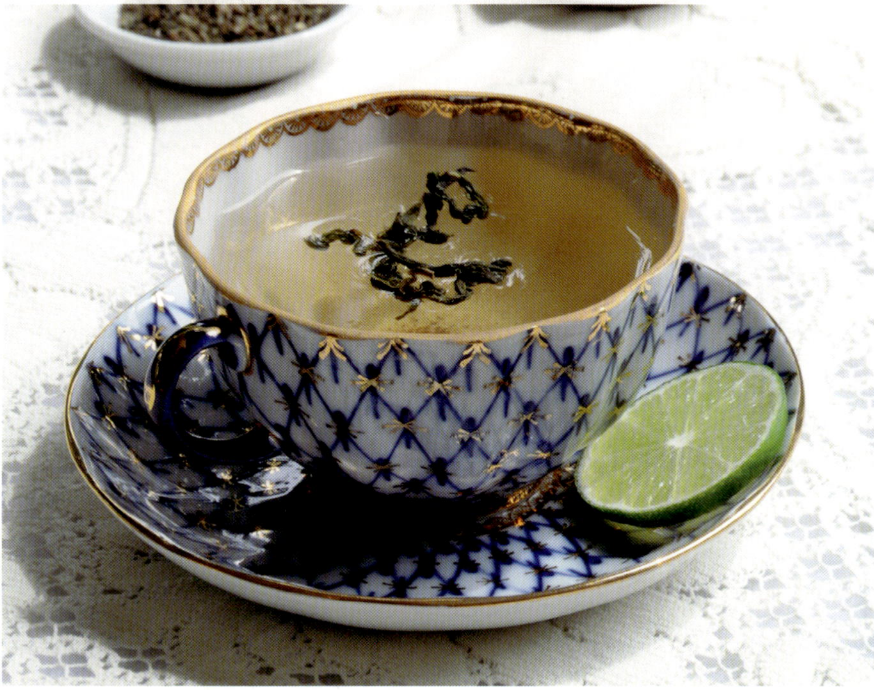

Ingredients

- 1 cup hot water
- ½ teaspoon Oolong tea (any variety)
- ¼ teaspoon spearmint, dried
- 1 allspice berry, crushed
- 1 slice lime

Directions

Garnish with a slice of lime and drink while hot. If you prefer a caffeine-free drink, substitute a peach-flavored teabag for the Oolong.

Serves 4

CURE FOR OVERINDULGENCE

Nothing makes a person feel and look more dragged out than the effects of overindulgence in alcohol. The following recipe may not be Jeeves', the consummate English butler's, cure, but it does a fair job. The recipe hails from the Mediterranean region and is "as old as the hills." Allegedly it also helps fan the flames of passion, increase fertility, and ensure success in all endeavors. A true cure-all! Persimmons were a highly prized fruit in days gone by, and I'm happy to see they are making something of a comeback.

Ingredients	Directions
½ cup persimmons, peeled and chopped	Blend; pour into glasses.
1 cup ginger tea, cooled	
1 pint barley water	
Honey to taste	

Weight Management

Lately, the media has been bombarding the public with disheartening statistics about the fattening of America and the many adults and children who are considered overweight or obese. While these sad facts may be true, the blame usually is laid squarely on the shoulders of the overweight individual. Finger-pointers contend that somehow it is the overweight person's fault that they eat too much and that they refuse to exercise.

Rarely does anybody note that the demanding, stress-inducing American lifestyle plays a large role. They often ignore the fact that the amount of processed foods with high salt and sugar content we consume because we lack the time to prepare meals from scratch exacerbates this problem. Environmental factors too complex to take up in this book also enter in.

People become depressed because their body image doesn't fit the ideal type flaunted onscreen or in magazines, so they eat even more to comfort themselves. Throughout this book I attempt to offer recipes that contain a minimum of salt and processed sugar. If you regularly consume some of these potions, your weight issues may begin to melt away on their own. In this section, I put forth a few suggestions for those of you who keenly feel the pressure to lose or gain weight to improve your body image. Keep in mind that no matter what your body looks like, it is yours, and it is beautiful.

Makes a batch

TO LOSE WEIGHT

Weight loss botanicals that have been consumed for centuries include celery, fennel, ginger, meadowsweet, onion, and green bean. (Believe it or not, the water left over from cooking green beans makes a superior weight loss tea.)

Here's another tip. Start your diet out right every morning by downing a tall glassful of water mixed with the juice of ½ lemon (no sweetener, please!). To help suppress your appetite, before eating, drink a steaming cupful of ginger tea flavored with cardamom and lemon. Stir with a cinnamon stick. If you don't have time to prepare this, a simple cup of green or black tea also works. Before bedtime, instead of snacking, drink a cupful of your favorite green tea sweetened with 1 teaspoon (no more!) of heather or clover honey.

Or, make up the following recipe.

Ingredients

- ¼ cup blackberry leaves
- ¼ cup alfalfa
- ¼ cup nettles
- 1 teaspoon buchu
- 1 teaspoon psyllium husks
- 1 teaspoon sage
- 1 teaspoon rose hips, crushed
- ¼ teaspoon juniper berries, crushed
- ¼ teaspoon licorice root powder

Directions

Because this recipe contains many ingredients, I find it convenient to put together a quantity to store. I add only ½ teaspoonful per cup of hot water. Use only dry ingredients for this recipe.

To Gain Weight

If, on the other hand, you'd like to bulk up, try adding ½ teaspoon of gentian root to any beverage infusion. You can also add kelp powder to just about any food. This seaweed is rich in nutrients and is a common food additive. Some nutritionally-minded folks use it in place of salt.

Now that you've made a big impression on the world around you, it's time to turn your attention closer to home, family, and friends.

Chapter 11

HOME SWEET HOME

Potions for Friendship and a Happy Home

Like many people, you've probably got tons of work commitments on top of a whirlwind social life. In fact, you have been so busy that perhaps you've neglected things on the home front somewhat–okay, maybe a lot. Time to reacquaint yourself with your home, family, and close friends. After all, isn't much of what you strive for in the outside world done so you can have a peaceful, prosperous domestic life?

Begin by taking a good look at where you live. Is everything neat and tidy and in its proper place? No cobwebs on the ceiling or dirt behind the door? No discarded items or trash lying about? If your home is well-ordered and sparkling, I offer you my congratulations. You can move on to the second part of this chapter that addresses relationships. However, if your place could use some sprucing up and the task seems overwhelming, read on for recipes to put you in the proper frame of mind to clean and organize.

Serves 2

FRIENDSHIP SMOOTHIE

Cement a budding friendship or strengthen the bond between you and a longtime friend with this delicious drink.

Ingredients

- ½ cup fresh or frozen currants (or ½ cup currant juice, which, I am happy to report, lately has become more readily available)
- ½ cup milk
- 2 tablespoons honey
- ½ teaspoon cinnamon powder
- ⅛ teaspoon clove powder (to nurture friendship)
- ½ cup ice cubes, more or less

Directions

Blend together and pour into 2 glasses, drink, relax, and enjoy each other's company.

Serves 1-2

Courage to CLEAN UP JUICE

They say that the condition of your home reflects your state of mind. Uh-oh! Does your place looks like a tornado hit it as mine does after the winter holidays are over? Are you having a hard time finding the motivation to clean your room, work area, home, or vehicle? Never fear. Prepare the following recipe in a juicer and all will be well.

Ingredients

- 1 small handful of fresh parsley*
- 2 stalks celery, cubed
- ½ cup fresh spinach, packed into the cup
- 4 carrots, cut into 2–3-inch lengths
- 1 small beet bulb, halved
- ¼ cup (more or less) of organic apple juice

Directions

Bunch up the parsley and spinach and guide them through the juicer with the celery, carrots, and beet. Add enough apple juice to sweeten the potion to taste, stir, and pour into a tall glass. Sip this energizing potion and—no excuses—get to work!

BOTANICALS WITH REPUTED SIMILAR EFFECTS

Fennel | Garlic | Onion | Vervain

* To the ancient Greeks, parsley symbolized victory

Serves 1-2

Dare to Organize TISANE

You've put your home back together. Give yourself a well-deserved pat on the back! But what about all those papers you threw in a heap on top of the desk or kitchen table, or squirreled away in a box to deal with later? The following beverage infusion will go a long way toward energizing you to tackle that daunting mound. It is made from botanicals that belong to the Virgo sign in astrology. Virgo is the organizer queen of the zodiac. Infuse the ingredients in 1 cup of hot water and drink it down.

Ingredients

- 1 teaspoon peppermint, cut and sifted
- ½ teaspoon fennel seed*
- ¼ teaspoon rosemary
- ¼ teaspoon whole cloves, crushed
- 2 pinches marjoram, cut and sifted
- 1 pinch dried skullcap (optional—this herb may only be available at an herb store or natural grocer. The recipe works fine without it.)

Directions

Make a beverage infusion from the ingredients following the directions from Chapter 4. If you're really serious about getting organized, wait for the tea to cool and add a shot of wheatgrass to spur you to action.

* For strength, heroism, and to stimulate courage

Serves 1

Where'd It Go? TEA

Photograph by C. Nathan Pulley Photography

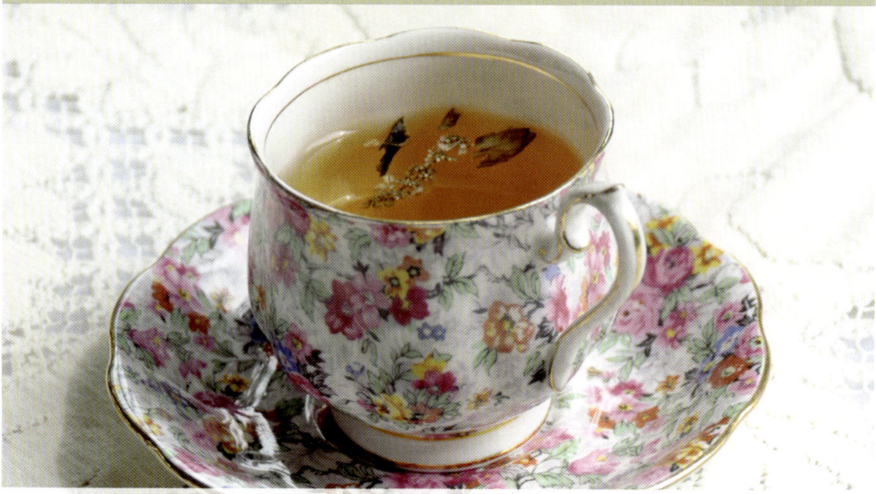

Even though you're more or less organized, occasionally something you need goes astray. Few things annoy me more than wasting precious time trolling around for an important misplaced item. My personal rule of thumb is to spend only five minutes searching for something inconsequential and no more than fifteen minutes on a really important item like my passport or tax documents. If, after fifteen minutes, you're in a royal snit, I suggest you take time out to prepare and drink this tea. The very act of preparation will help still your mind to the point that the place of concealment will almost certainly reveal itself to you.

Ingredients

- ½ teaspoon gunpowder green tea (or 1 teabag)
- ¼ teaspoon peppermint
- ¼ teaspoon anise

Directions

While the infusion steeps, thoroughly clean the kitchen table, or wherever you eat. Put away all the papers and other junk that has accumulated there. When the infusion is ready, sit at the table, ground and center yourself, and sip the tea. Soon ideas will come to you about where to look for the missing article. Do not force an idea. Let your stream of consciousness flow until it leads you to the lost item. Refrain from acting on impulse and leisurely finish your tea. Now rise and go directly to the object.

If you still are having trouble locating that pesky document, return to the teacup, drain away any droplets of water that still may be clinging to the bottoms or sides, and see if you can discern in the leaves an image of the place where the missing paper is buried. Gunpowder green tea renders a few bold images, so it is good for answering simple questions such as "Where is blankety-blank hiding?" For more tips on reading the leaves, see the section in Chapter 5 of this book on coffee ground reading. Many of the same techniques apply to tealeaf reading.

Serves 2-4

Bless and Protect This Home PASTA SAUCE

Photograph by C. Nathan Pulley Photography

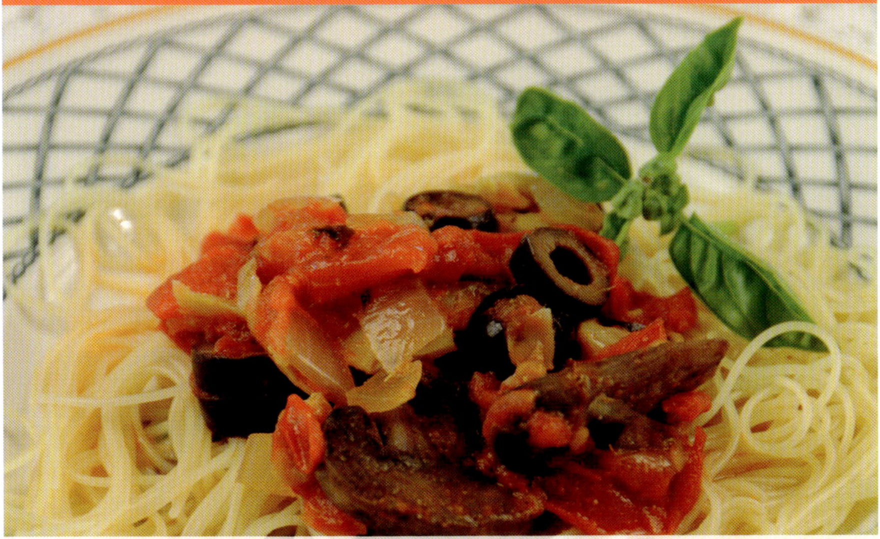

Everything in your house is nestled in its proper place–well, nearly everything. Your space is sparkling like a summer morning. Now is the perfect time to gather relatives and friends around the dinner table to bless your home. Nothing spells comfort and blessings like an old-fashioned spaghetti dinner. The following pasta recipe, which relies on many fresh ingredients, is one of my favorites.

Ingredients

- 1 small jar marinated artichoke hearts
- ½ onion, diced
- 1 cup mushrooms, sliced
- 2 garlic cloves, diced
- ¼ cup jicama, diced (optional)
- 4 tomatoes, diced
- 1 tablespoon fresh basil, chopped
- 1 tablespoon fresh parsley, chopped
- Salt and pepper to taste
- 1 small can (2 oz.) green olives, sliced

Directions

Remove the artichoke hearts from the jar, dice, and set aside. Use the oil from the jar to sauté the onion, mushrooms, garlic, and jicama. Add the tomatoes, basil, and parsley. Bring to a boil and cook uncovered for 15 minutes. Salt and pepper to taste. Lower the heat; cover, and simmer until the mixture thickens, for at least another 10 minutes. Before serving, add olive slices and stir.

Serve it over spinach noodles or angel hair pasta with a side salad and grape juice or red wine. Grape drinks are alleged to foster cordiality. (See photo at beginning of chapter.)

This recipe is reputed to have the added benefit of increasing male virility. *Ciao* Viagra!

Serves the home only (not for drinking)

Bless My Home and Keep It Safe SPRINKLING TEA

This is the only recipe in this book not meant to be consumed. Although all of the ingredients are edible, the frankincense will make it taste bitter. The idea of this potion is to give your home, rather than you, a good drink.

Ingredients

- 4 cups water
- 2 teaspoons chamomile
- 1 teaspoon lemon balm
- 1 teaspoon lemon verbena
- 1 teaspoon lavender flowers
- 1 teaspoon bayberry bark
- ½ teaspoon basil
- ¼ teaspoon frankincense powder

Directions

Combine all of the ingredients in a saucepan and boil until the liquid has reduced to approximately 3 cups. Strain away the botanicals, and set aside. Sprinkle the water through all parts of the house, especially in the corners of rooms, on window ledges, doorways, and over the threshold.

For added effect, if you live in a house with a door to the outside, you can strew the leftover herbs around the front door and on the walk leading to the house. Perhaps you live in an apartment and can't do this, but you may have a parking space on the street or in a garage. If so, place the herbs there (especially on the tires of your car). They will help bless and protect you in your vehicle, which can be considered as your home away from home.

Your home is now thoroughly blessed, so let's move on to blessing our intimate relationships.

Serves 2

Let's Not Bicker TISANE

Tired of squabbling with family, colleagues, or friends? To restore amity to your relationships, make a beverage infusion as follows:

Ingredients	Directions
2 cups hot water 1 teaspoon chamomile flowers, dried ½ teaspoon hibiscus flowers, dried 1 olive leaf, dried and crushed Pinch dill weed Organic sugar to taste	Usually, I don't recommend sugar in teas or herbal infusions, but since sugar is alleged to sweeten one's humor, in this case I say, "Go for it." Combine all of the ingredients except the sugar and add the hot water. Steep for three minutes or more. Pour the liquid through a strainer into 2 china teacups, and sweeten to taste. While both of you sip the brew, seek to identify common ground. Calmly discuss points of friction and how to harmonize your differences.

OTHER INGREDIENTS APPROPRIATE FOR POTIONS TO HARMONIZE RELATIONSHIPS OR ATMOSPHERES OF A PLACE (SUCH AS A HAUNTED HOUSE)

Clove
Flax
Horehound
Kava-kava
Thyme

Now that your living space is gleaming like a bright star and your nearest and dearest have gathered around, the next chapter will focus on your physical body.

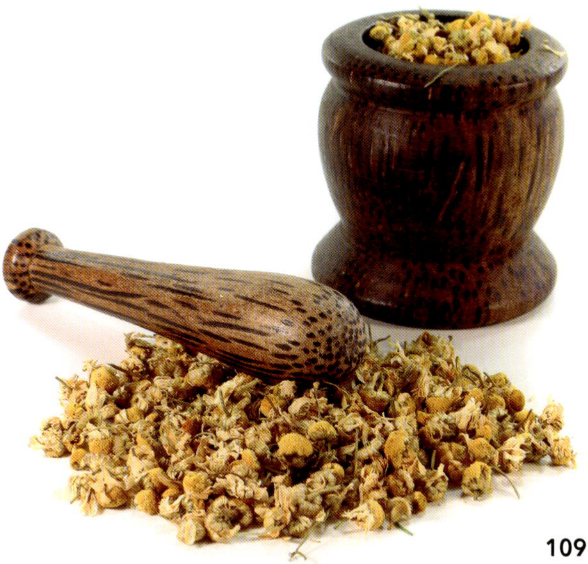

Chapter 12

THE BEST YOU CAN BE

Potions for Physical and Mental Health

In this chapter you'll find ideas for potions to nurture your physical and mental bodies. To keep yourself in tiptop shape, here are some general potion ingredients: carrot, coriander, ginger, grapefruit, honey, lemon, mustard, papaya, plum, potato, pumpkin, rosemary. For specific recipes, read on.

Serves 1

Front and Center TEA

I often hear people complain that they fear they may be falling out of balance, mentally, emotionally, and physically. These folks spend a lot of time and energy on methods for centering and grounding such as yoga, Pilates, and breathing exercises. Although such remedies can be useful, I also believe that if you want to get back into equilibrium, you need to live right. This means you should never desire bad things to befall others or harm another being—human or animal. Respect life; be a giving person. This attitude will go a long way toward balancing body, mind, and spirit.

Here's a simple infusion tailor-made to plant your feet firmly on the ground.

Ingredients

- 1 cup hot water
- ¼ teaspoon lavender
- ¼ teaspoon rose hips, crushed
- ½ teaspoon pink rose petals, fresh, if possible

Directions

Infuse the formula in 1 cup of hot water and drink.

OTHER BOTANICALS FOR CENTERING AND GROUNDING:

Caraway seed (for self-control)
Celery leaf and seed
Hibiscus
Maidenhair
Peppermint
Valerian

Serves 2

Lullaby TEA

First things first! To stay fit, trim, and alert, you need to get a good night's rest every night. Unfortunately, this is easier said than done. The stresses and worries of contemporary life can interfere with normal sleep patterns. The following potion is designed to lull you into peaceful slumber without making you feel groggy the following day.

Ingredients

- ½ teaspoon green tea (any variety, or 1 green teabag)
- ½ teaspoon chamomile flowers, dried
- ¼ teaspoon hops flowers, dried
- ¼ teaspoon valerian root, dried and diced
- ¼ teaspoon lemon catnip tea (optional)*

Directions

This recipe renders at least 2 cups. If you don't want to prepare it from scratch every night, multiply the amounts and store the dry blend in an airtight container. Use ½ teaspoon per cup of hot tea.

By the way, the hops in the above potion are purported to prevent nightmares. Maybe that's why many people enjoy drinking beer—for its medicinal value, of course!

OTHER HERBS TRADITIONALLY HELD TO INDUCE A GOOD NIGHT'S REST

Agrimony

COWSLIP (LATELY THIS BOTANICAL HAS BEEN ON THE ENDANGERED SPECIES LIST, SO PLEASE CHECK TO SEE IF IT'S STILL THERE BEFORE BUYING)

Dill
Feverfew
Olive leaf
Motherwort
Poppy seed (for pleasant dreams)

* The San Francisco Herb Company (www.sfherbco.com) sells a good lemon-catnip tea.

Serves 4

Can't Afford to Get Sick BORSCHT

Rather than battle a cold, it is best not to fall ill in the first place. Remember earlier when I mentioned that red liquids are associated with good health? This crimson-colored recipe will help combat all kinds of crud—a highly technical term for colds and flu, especially those that creep around during the winter months. As an added bonus, this soup tastes even better on the second day and can be served hot or cold.

Ingredients

- 3–4 medium beets, peeled and shredded
- 4 cups vegetable stock
- ¼ cup vinegar
- 1 tablespoon honey
- 1 teaspoon dried sage or 4 fresh sage leaves, chopped
- 2 teaspoons tamari sauce
- ¼ medium cabbage, shredded
- ½ cup tomato juice
- Plain yogurt or sour cream for garnish

Directions

Combine the beets and stock in a big pot and cook covered over low heat until the beets are tender, approximately 30 minutes. Add the honey, vinegar, tamari, and cabbage. Cover, and cook until the cabbage begins to soften, for 10 minutes or so. Stir in the tomato juice and cook until well blended. Cool the mixture and put it through a blender until smooth. If desired, reheat the soup to serve it hot. Garnish with plain yogurt or sour cream.

Serves 1

Can't Afford to Get Sick TISANE

If you would rather not drink soup, here's another "ounce of prevention" recipe to take as a beverage infusion every morning during the flu season.

Ingredients

- 1 cup hot water
- ½ teaspoon fresh sage leaves, chopped
- ¼ teaspoon angelica root, chopped
- ¼ teaspoon feverfew flowers
- 2 pinches elecampane herb, cut and sifted
- Two pinches ginseng powder

Directions

Make a beverage infusion from the ingredients as explained in Chapter 4. Remember to strain away the botanicals before drinking.

Serves 2

Banish Depression and Melancholy HOT COCOA TEA

A person's state of health often depends on the mental and emotional frame of mind. When you feel gloomy or despondent, you may leave yourself open for illness to grab a foothold. Lift your spirits with this appetizing tea. Drink it anytime you feel dejection closing in.

Ingredients

- 1 cup water
- 1 green teabag (any kind or brand will do. I favor Sencha) or 1 Lady Grey black teabag
- 1 cup fat-free milk
- 1 tablespoon unsweetened cocoa
- 1 tablespoon demerara or turbinado sugar (or sweeten to taste)
- ½ teaspoon vanilla extract
- ¼ teaspoon almond extract
- ⅛ teaspoon cinnamon, ground
- ⅛ teaspoon ginger, ground
- ⅛ teaspoon allspice, ground

Directions

Bring the water to a boil in a saucepan. Remove the saucepan from the heat; add the teabag and steep for 3–5 minutes. While waiting for the tea to steep, in a separate saucepan, heat the milk with the rest of the ingredients until the mixture boils, stirring constantly. When the tea has steeped, remove the bag, add the tea to the milk, and stir well. Pour into mugs and drink immediately.

GENERAL DISPOSITION BRIGHTENERS:

Blessed thistle
Borage
Cardamom
Chamomile
Chocolate
Lemon
Lemon balm
Motherwort
Yarrow

Do You Want to Live Forever?

People from all cultures over time have ardently sought the magic bullet to restore youth and virility and to extend their lifespans. A case in point are the magicians of the Renaissance. They developed many health potions in the course of their quest for the elixir of life. Their research resulted in a new kind of medical treatment that eventually became known as homeopathy. In another example, Spanish Conquistador Ponce de León searched high and low for the Fountain of Youth. Although he never found it, he ended up discovering Florida, which many people even today consider to be a true tropical paradise.

A daily glass of tomato juice has long been prescribed by herbalists as a potion to extend the lifespan. Other botanicals with a similar reputation include: alfalfa, garlic, ginseng, lady's mantle, lemon, life everlasting, lemon balm, pear, and plum. Here are a couple of potions that take advantage of reputed life-enhancing ingredients. You might also want to turn to Appendix A on page 152 to read about the nutritional virtues of tomatoes, pears, and raspberries that help support the life-extension claims for these recipes.

Serves 4

Cream of Fresh TOMATO SOUP

Canned tomato soup can't hold a candle to this fresh alternative. Simply sniffing and tasting this rich soup, I believe can add years to your life. This is one of my favorite recipes.

Ingredients

- 2 ripe tomatoes, chopped
- ¼ cup green onion, chopped
- 1 bay leaf (for victory)
- 2 tablespoons butter
- 2 tablespoons all-purpose flour
- ¼ teaspoon salt
- 2 cups milk
- Salt and pepper to taste
- Parsley, green onion, or grated cheddar cheese for garnish

Directions

In a saucepan, simmer the tomato, onion, and bay on very low heat for 10 minutes. (The juice from the tomato should keep the mixture from catching on, but if it threatens to burn add a tablespoon or two of water.) Sieve, and set aside. In the same saucepan, melt the butter and stir in the flour and salt. Add the milk, and cook over low heat, stirring constantly until mixture thickens. Slowly stir in the hot tomato mixture until blended; salt and pepper to taste. Garnish with fresh parsley, green onion, or grated cheddar cheese, if desired.

Serves 2

Life Everlasting JUICE

All of the ingredients in this recipe are purported to help a person live a long, healthy life.

Ingredients

- 2 pears, cut into eighths
- 1 cup raspberries
- 1 teaspoon lady's mantle (optional)
- 10 drops ginseng extract (or 1 ginseng teabag or 1 packet freeze-dried ginseng—I like the Prince of Peace brand, but use your favorite.)
- 1 tablespoon protein powder
- Water
- Sprig of peppermint for garnish

Directions

Alternate layers of pears and raspberries in the juicer and process well after each addition. Add the rest of the ingredients and blend well. Add water until you get the consistency you wish. Pour into glasses and garnish with sprigs of fresh peppermint before serving.

Serves 3-4 (depending on portion)

Prevent an Accident SMOOTHIE

Help prevent sports accidents and injuries and energize yourself by drinking the following potion before you begin any competition.

Ingredients

- ½ cup pineapple juice
- ½ cup peach nectar
- ¾ cup peaches, peeled, pitted, and diced
- ¾ cup fresh pineapple, peeled and diced (or ¾ cup canned)
- 1 cup low fat peach frozen yogurt
- ½ teaspoon motherwort, cut and sifted (for protection)
- ¼ teaspoon bay leaf powder (for protection)
- 1 sprig fresh monarda mint (or any kind of mint for increased energy), chopped

Directions

Mix the ingredients in a blender on low speed until blended. Pick up speed until the mixture is smooth. Garnish with a slice of peach and a sprig of mint. Monarda has the peppery taste of bergamot, a key ingredient of Earl Grey tea, but peppermint or spearmint will do just as nicely.

Serves 4

Competitive Edge SPINACH SOUP

This recipe, handed down to me from my mother, is messy to prepare but mouth-watering to drink. And, as it does for Popeye, the spinach will fortify you to maintain that competitive edge.

Ingredients

- 1 teaspoon salt
- 3 10-ounce packages frozen spinach
- 4 cups water, split
- 2 teaspoons chicken broth granules
- 2 large potatoes, cubed
- 2 tablespoons butter
- 1 large onion, finely chopped
- 1 stick (¼ pound) butter
- ½ cup sour cream
- Salt and pepper to taste

Directions

In a saucepan, add the salt to the first 2 cups of water, then the spinach; cook until tender. Drain the water into a large pot, and set aside the spinach. Add 1 to 2 teaspoons of chicken broth granules to the hot water and dissolve.

In the meantime, in another saucepan, cook the potatoes in the remaining 2 cups water until tender. Add 2 tablespoons of butter and mash.

Melt the stick of butter in a frying pan, add the onion, and cook until the onion is transparent, but not brown.

Place the cooked onion and butter mixture and enough spinach in a blender until the blender is approximately half full, and blend. Now blend in the rest of the spinach.

Put this mixture into the pot of spinach-chicken broth and fold in the mashed potatoes.

Heat gently; when heated, add the sour cream. Add salt and pepper to taste. Pour the soup into bowls and enjoy with a hearty hunk of bread and butter (artisan black olive bread is one of my favorites). And congratulations for mastering this complex recipe!

Body Tune-Up and Tone-Up Juice

For an all-around body toner, a mixture of carrot juice and coconut water with a few fresh sprigs of added parsley or fennel is hard to beat.

Carrots contain beta carotene and the coconut water is chock full of potassium. And both are low-calorie.

Serves 2

POTION to Heal the Environment

Finally, as you're enlivening your body, you might give a thought to how to improve the physical condition of the planet. Ideally, the following libation should accompany a solo or group pledge to clean, protect, and preserve the environment. It is designed to help steady your resolve and spur you to action.

Ingredients	Directions
1½ cups mango juice	Combine the ingredients in a blender and blend well.
12 strawberries	
½ peach, sliced	
¼ teaspoon cardamom	

Peace on Earth and goodwill to all!

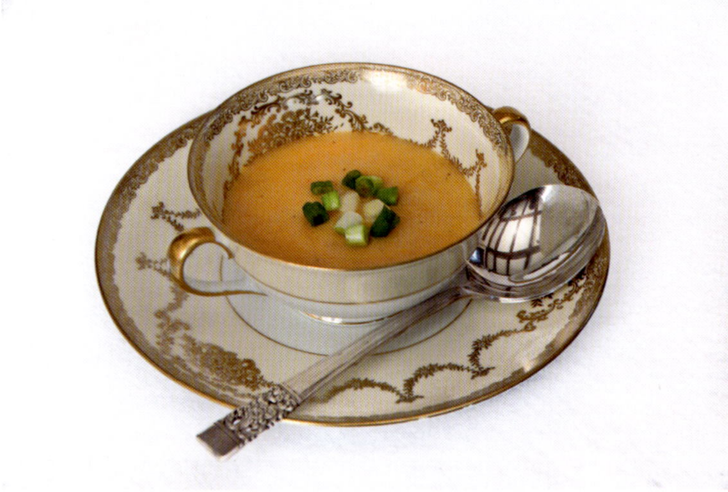

Cream of Fresh Tomato Soup. **(Recipe on page 114.)**

Chapter 13

USING YOUR NUT

Potions for Intellectual Pursuits and Goals

I don't have a magic pill that will enable you to peer beyond the boundaries of our universe, much less raise your IQ to 200. What I can offer in this chapter are potions to help you achieve your intellectual goals and pursuits. Whether you are a student cramming for finals, a realtor hopefully prepping to pass the estate board exam, an employee desiring to learn more about a chosen field, or a senior striving to sharpen what world-renowned mystery writer Agatha Christie's famous detective Hercule Poirot calls "the little gray cells"–your intellect–first and foremost, you'll want to perfect your study habits. What more agreeable way to do it than with the aid of the following potion?

Serves 2

Study Better SMOOTHIE

Ingredients

- 1–2 tablespoons low-fat milk
- 3 tablespoons chocolate syrup
- 1 tablespoon coconut, shredded
- 1 banana, sliced
- 2 cups vanilla low-fat frozen yogurt
- ½ teaspoon cinnamon
- ¼ teaspoon almond extract

Directions

Place the ingredients in a blender and mix on low speed until blended. Continue blending, gradually increasing speed until the mixture is smooth. Pour into glasses and sprinkle with unsweetened cocoa powder. Garnish with a bright red maraschino cherry to fire you up to crack the books. Share this delight with your study partner. Who says studying is boring?

OTHER BOTANICALS CLAIMED TO GIVE YOU THAT STUDY HALL EDGE:

Lavender Broccoli Basil

Photograph by C. Nathan Pulley Photography

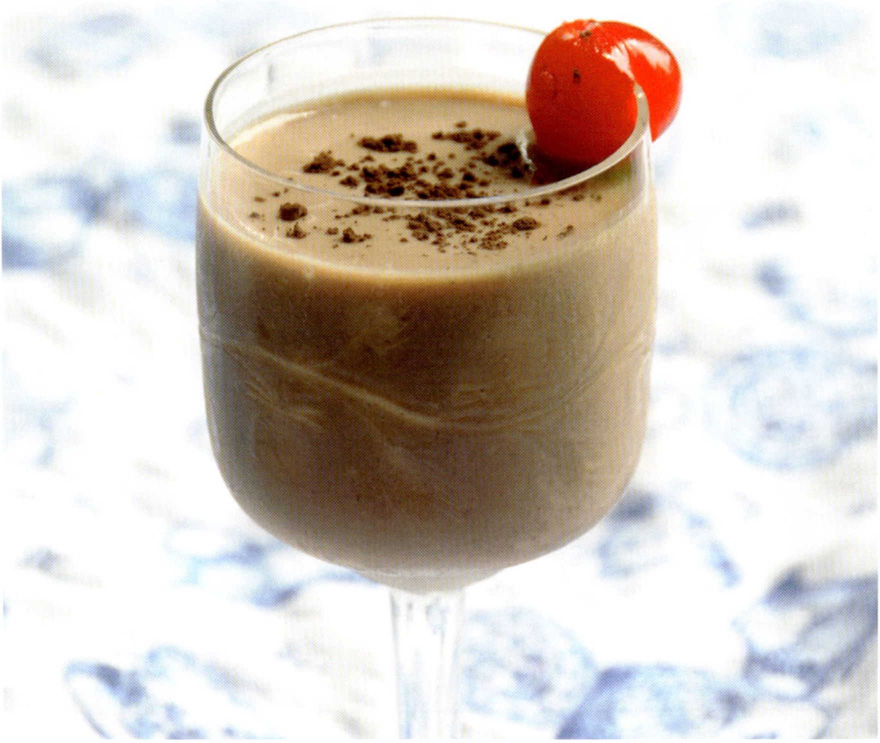

Serves 1-2

Ace That Test MOCHA MALT

Whether you're burning the midnight oil for a biology final, sweating over a CPA certification, learning a foreign language because you're going abroad on holiday, or simply working to finish your taxes on time, top off your session with this delicious mocha malt. It will restore those little gray cells and relax and refresh you.

Ingredients

- 1 cup low fat frozen vanilla yogurt
- ½ cup low fat milk
- 1 tablespoon instant malted milk powder
- 1 tablespoon instant Swiss-style coffee powder

Directions

Combine the ingredients in a blender. Cover and blend until smooth. Pour into a tall glass and drink up. Now march into the exam room and knock 'em dead with your knowledge and expertise.

BOTANICALS WITH SIMILAR REPUTED QUALITIES:

Bay (for victory)

Kinnickinnick (for improved mental faculties)

Life everlasting and rosemary (for enhanced memory)

Enhance Your Concentration Abilities

Having trouble concentrating? Perhaps you've got too many distractions running interference. Or maybe your interest in the subject is slim. But, hey, you've got to get whatever it is done, and the sooner you finish, the sooner you'll be free to move on to greener pastures. So turn off your mobile device, promise yourself you won't text or answer any emails until the task is complete, and retire to a quiet place where you can think and work undisturbed.

To concentrate better, you will want to polish your powers of visualization, for visualization and concentration go hand-in-hand. My advice in this area is to not try to focus your attention by force of will. You will tire easily, and eventually lose the ability to keep your mind on the subject. Start by relaxing, but stay alert. The Mocha Malt recipe that follows this section will help you achieve this balanced frame of mind.

Next, create some positive images and affirmations to dwell on rather than negative ones. What I mean by this is don't tell yourself, "I need to concentrate to achieve this or my life is over." Affirm instead, "The way is clear for me to focus on the goal that I know will bring me success."

Inhale positive images and exhale negative ones. Before retiring at night, conjure to your mind's eye the key images you constructed and say your affirmations aloud. Eat green foods and drink plenty of water. If you are concocting a complex potion merely as an excuse to procrastinate, save time and buy prepared juices. The Naked and Odwalla brands as well as V-8 Fusion, among others, offer dynamite healthy green fare.

If, on the other hand, you desire to try your hand at preparing a personalized concentration potion, here are some suggestions for botanicals believed to help fix your attention and increase your understanding of situations:

- Allspice
- Almond
- Artichoke
- Basil
- Broccoli
- Celery seed and stalk
- Cinnamon
- Dill seed boiled in red wine (a centuries-old potion)
- Eyebright
- Garlic
- Lavender
- Mango
- Meadowsweet
- Motherwort
- Mustard
- Sage
- Salt
- Spikenard (known as "the consummate brain food")
- Strawberry

For sample recipes, read on.

Serves 6

Make the Right Choice
BEAN SOUP

Part of achieving your aims involves choosing which goals are worth the effort. Only then can you set targets appropriate to your situation.

A pleasant way to contemplate your choices is over a bowl of fragrant fifteen-bean soup. In my pre-published mystery novel, *Scent of Murder*, my main character's spirit granny whips up a steaming pot of this aromatic soup to help the amateur sleuth ferret out the murderer's true identity. Your goal may not be as dramatic. Nonetheless, it is important to you and deserves at least one bowlful of this soup to aid your contemplation.

Ingredients

- 1 8-ounce bag of fifteen beans
- 1 leek, chopped
- ½ cup celery, diced
- 1 carrot, diced
- 2 cloves garlic, pressed
- 1 teaspoon fresh basil
- 1 teaspoon fennel seeds (helps resolve problems)
- 1 bay leaf
- 2 tablespoons bacon, fried and crumbled (or 2 tablespoons "faux" bacon made from soy)
- Shredded cheddar or mild white cheese for garnish

Directions

Prepare the contents of a small bag (8 ounces) of fifteen-bean soup by washing the beans and soaking them overnight in salted water. In the morning, strain away the water, wash the beans again, and place them in a pot along with 6 cups of water. Bring the beans and water to a boil and add the rest of the ingredients, salt and pepper to taste. (For those who practice divination, pepper is alleged to send correct answers from Spirit.)

Simmer until the beans soften. Remove the bay leaf before serving; garnish with shredded cheddar or mild white cheese, such as farmer's cheese, *queso de Oaxaca*, or *queso fresco*.

BOTANICALS TO HELP YOU MAKE RIGHT DECISIONS

Apple
Bay
Fennel
Leek
Pepper

Serves 6-8 (depending on whether you pour it over a main dish or a dessert)

Top Drawer PLUM SAUCE

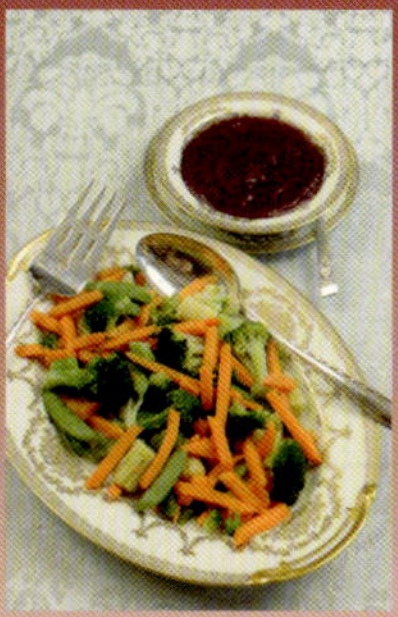

The ancient Chinese prized the pretty purple plum for the fruit's alleged ability to slow aging and confer the best of health and wisdom. For you high achievers who want to stay in first-class form, here's a delicious recipe for plum sauce. Pour it over ice cream or use as a sauce for Oriental vegetables, chicken, beef, or pork. The recipe delivers a double wallop of intelligence because it also includes apple, which according to the ancient Celts, also bestows wisdom.

Ingredients

- 1 pound fresh plums, pitted and quartered
- 1 cup apples, peeled, cored, and quartered
- 3 tablespoons water
- ½ cup apricot preserves
- ½ cup pineapple, crushed
- Organic brown sugar, to taste
- 1 tablespoon vinegar
- ½ teaspoon ginger
- ½ teaspoon garlic
- ½ teaspoon hot pepper (cayenne, hot banana, jalapeño, serrano, etc.)

Directions

Combine the plums, apples, and water in a large saucepan. Cover and cook over medium-low heat for 10 minutes until the fruit is soft, stirring occasionally. Let cool for 15 minutes, and puree in a food processor or blender. Add remaining ingredients, blending well. Chill mixture for at least 2 hours to let the flavors intermingle before eating.

OTHER BOTANICALS ALLEGED TO KEEP THOSE SYNAPSES FIRING

Allspice
Berry
Cinnamon
Fennel
Lavender
Sage
Spearmint
Thyme

In the next chapter, you'll learn to communicate to others all of the celebrated knowledge you've just acquired from learning to use your nut.

Chapter 14

SAY WHAT?

Potions for Communication and Travel

Keep a Secret TEA

Serves 2 cups

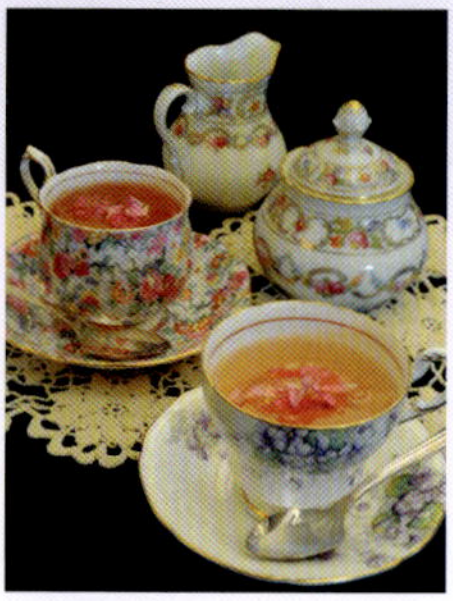

Now that you are renowned for your intelligence, knowledge, wisdom, and perky personality, you may find that people are sharing their most closely guarded secrets. To help you remain loyal and keep confidences, share this cup of tea with your trusted comrade.

Ingredients

- 2 cups water
- 1 teaspoon Darjeeling tea
- ½ teaspoon lavender flowers, dried
- ½ teaspoon rose petals, fresh (or ½ teaspoon dried)

Directions

Boil the water; let it cool for 2 minutes. Add the dry ingredients and steep for 2–3 more minutes. Strain away the botanicals and pour the scented tea into 2 cups and serve.

Following are more recipes to facilitate different kinds of communication scenarios.

Serves 1

Come Together INFUSION

If you've ever tried to bring together a group of like-minded individuals and ended up frustrated from wrestling to coordinate everyone's busy schedules, this is the potion for you. Prepare a steaming cup of the following herbal infusion. After consuming it, go to your computer, phone, or mobile device, and contact everyone with the schedule that they all surely will be able to accommodate.

You can also drink this tea prior to leaving to attend a religious, social, business, or professional group, or other potential venue to meet people of your particular orientation and interests. This tisane also works well when you desire to meet up with like-minded individuals while traveling.

Ingredients

- 1 cup hot water
- ½ teaspoon Rooibos (or 1 Rooibos teabag)
- ½ teaspoon hibiscus flowers, dried
- ¼ teaspoon fresh gingerroot, grated
- ¼ bay leaf, crushed (or 2 pinches bay leaf powder)

Directions

If you can't find fresh gingerroot while on the road, use a pinch or two of powdered ginger. Also hibiscus flowers can often be found in teabag form.

Serves 2

Failure to Communicate TEA FIX

If you've tried the prior recipes but still are having trouble getting your ideas across, this tea will help ease the path toward understanding.

Ingredients

- 2 cups hot water
- 1 teaspoon Lapsang Souchong tea (a smoky-tasting black tea)
- ½ teaspoon elder flowers
- ½ teaspoon borage flowers
- ¼ teaspoon galangal root, cut
- ¼ teaspoon rosemary

Directions

Infuse the ingredients together for 3 minutes before drinking. Since this recipe renders 2 cups of tea, I suggest you share it with the person with whom you wish to communicate.

Serves 1

Communicate Through the Arts or Internet TISANE

Whether you choose to express yourself through music, writing, art, drama, or dance, shine in speech class, blog on the Internet, hobnob with fairies, spirits, or even with ghosts, everything boils down to communication. The following beverage infusion is alleged to open your path to effective artistic self-expression.

Ingredients

- 1 cup hot water
- ½ teaspoon lemon balm, cut and sifted
- ½ teaspoon dried lemon peel
- ½ teaspoon dried orange peel
- Pinch of cinnamon

Directions

Steep the ingredients for 3–4 minutes, sieve and drink. It tastes delicious iced or hot.

Serves 4

Listen Up! MUSHROOM SOUP

Have you ever struggled to get your voice heard or convince someone to see your point of view at home, work, school, or in the neighborhood? Nudge yourself over the communications hurdle by drinking this soup on the evening before the big encounter.

Ingredients

- 1 cup water
- 1 teaspoon salt
- ½ teaspoon ground black pepper
- 1 chicken bouillon cube
- 4 tablespoons butter, split
- 1 pound fresh mushrooms, sliced, split
- 2 teaspoons lemon juice
- 1 leek, chopped
- 2 carrots, sliced
- 2 tablespoons flour
- 2 cups milk
- 2 tablespoons dry sherry
- 2 teaspoons fresh dill, chopped (or ½ teaspoon dried) for garnish, if desired

Directions

Heat the water to boiling and dissolve the bouillon cube. Add salt and pepper and set aside. In a saucepan, melt the butter over medium heat. Add the mushrooms and lemon juice; cook until mushrooms are just tender. Set aside in a bowl.

Melt the remaining butter in a pot. Add the leeks and carrots; sauté for 5 minutes. Stir in the flour until blended; then stir in the milk, mushrooms, prepared water, and sherry. Reheat and serve. Garnish with fresh dill, if desired.

Serves 1

Commune with Nature
STRAWBERRY JUICE

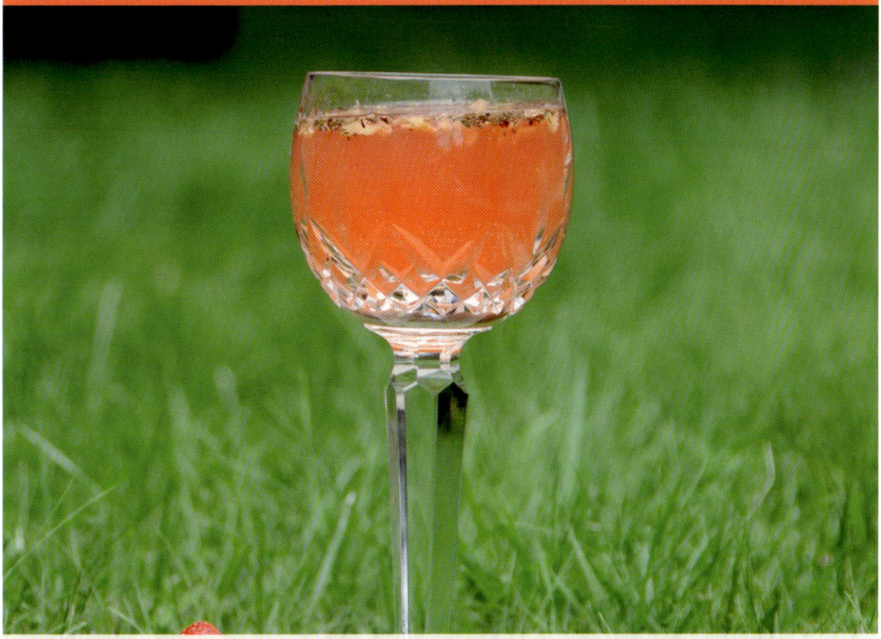

Photograph by C. Nathan Pulley Photography

An aspect of communication that many of us don't often think about is communication with the natural world around us. The next time you take a walk in a forest, botanical garden, on the beach, through a field, or even in your own backyard, bring along a thermos full of the following juice. It's simple to make but sweetly refreshing. Folklore has it that this juice also facilitates contact and communication between humans and the delightful mythical elemental creatures known as fairies.

Ingredients

- 12 strawberries (or one 12-ounce can strawberry juice from the grocery)
- 3 strawberries, sliced
- ½ teaspoon gingerroot, fresh
- ½ teaspoon chipped thyme, chopped
- Honey, to taste

Directions

Juice a glassful (approximately 12) fresh strawberries or buy strawberry juice from the grocery store. Grate approximately ½ teaspoonful of fresh gingerroot into the thermos and add ½ teaspoon of fresh chopped thyme. (If you're using dried thyme, reduce the amount to ¼ teaspoon.) Sweeten to taste with honey (one of the fairies' alleged favorite foods), garnish with sliced strawberries, and shake well before drinking. If you want to make this potion more liquid, add carbonated water until you get the desired consistency.

Serves 2

Talk to the Animals TEA

Now that I've got you tramping around out in the wild, you might want to try the following infusion to help understand the language and communicate with wildlife. It is alleged to work equally well with domestic animal and pets. The tea also facilitates meditation to discover your personal power or totem animal. I happened to drink this tea early one morning last winter.

Ingredients

- 2 cups hot water
- 1 teaspoon green tea, or 2 green teabags
- 1 teaspoon dandelion leaves
- ½ teaspoon elecampane
- ¼ teaspoon spikenard
- ¼ teaspoon valerian
- ¼ teaspoon caraway
- Pinch of horehound

Directions

Infuse the botanicals and let me know what kind of wildlife shows up in your garden.

Travel

When you travel domestically or abroad, either alone, or with companions, you may want and need to reach out to those around you. Although learning to speak the language of the country is helpful, you really don't need to talk in order to communicate effectively. And this nugget of advice comes from a former professor of Portuguese and Spanish and intercultural trainer—me!

I am reminded of the time when the company I worked for asked me to invite for dinner two Japanese men who were learning to speak English at the center. These fellows had very minimal English skills, and I spoke only three words of Japanese. So I invited an affable American friend to join us.

After a disastrous beginning, when we all struggled to communicate even the most basic pleasantries, our friend hit on a scheme. Somehow, through a variety of pantomime gestures, he got across the idea of the sound English-speakers make to refer to a dog—"bow-wow." The Japanese students indicated the sound they make for a dog in their language. After imitating cats, birds, sheep, horses, cows and a whole barnyard of creatures in both languages, our gathering dissolved into gales of laughter. A good time was had by all without ever having to tussle with opinions on world politics or other weighty matters.

The sort of interaction described above is a form of non-verbal communication known as paralinguistic activity. To interact effectively with others, no matter where they come from, I suggest you become a keen observer of other people's behaviors and modify your own outward behavior accordingly.

It is a known fact that sixty to seventy percent of what we communicate is through nonverbal expression. Nonverbal behavior includes posture, style of dress, the physical distance people stand from each other, how they walk, their facial expressions and tone of voice, eye movements, and many other activities. Bear this in mind when attempting to communicate with others away from your comfort zone.

Spearmint, Peppermint, Cinnamon, and Clove for Intercultural Communication

It can be difficult to concoct potions when you are away from your kitchen, so in this section I will not suggest specific recipes. If you want to facilitate communication with others while away from home, you might want to look for teas or tisanes that include spearmint, peppermint, cinnamon, and clove. All of these botanicals are commonly found worldwide. Order the tisane when you dine at a café or restaurant. You can also choose something to eat that contains these herbs as well as cinnamon and clove. Many desserts and sauces include at least one ingredient.

Spearmint and peppermint offer the added benefit of settling your stomach. This certainly is a plus when traveling, especially when you find yourself experimenting with unfamiliar foods in unaccustomed settings. As I mentioned in an earlier chapter, cinnamon and clove, which possess antibacterial properties, will help kill the pesky bacteria foreign to your digestive system.

If you're concerned about personal safety when traveling, you will find recipes in Chapter 16. Also when on the road, I suggest you go for teas, foods, sauces–anything edible or drinkable–that contain artichoke, chamomile, cranberry, grapefruit, grapes (think red wine, also celebrated for its resveratrol content, which is good for the heart), hops (think beer), potatoes, and rosemary.

Serves 1

Bon Voyage JUICE

Before departing on your journey, treat yourself to the following juice to get communications off on the right foot.

Ingredients

- 1 cup mango, diced
- ½ cup peaches
- ½ cup pineapple
- ¼ teaspoon allspice

Directions

Blend the ingredients in your juicer. If you prefer a beverage with alcohol, add grenadine to taste.

Chapter 15

INNER JOURNEYS

Potions for the Spiritual and Creative Side of Life

Recent surveys in national newspapers and magazines note that Americans are becoming increasingly interested in spiritual matters. Whether this is a reaction to the emphasis on materialism in contemporary society or a new millennium phenomenon linked to the Age of Aquarius is hard to tell. Fact is, more people are buying books and CDs on spirituality, attending religious meetings, participating in spiritually oriented seminars and the like than ever before.

Fast Food Spirituality

One aspect of modern American society is our enjoyment of and insistence on instant service. Stores are open twenty-four hours a day. We order merchandise online anytime we feel like it. We are enthralled watching instant replay at televised athletic events and stream entertainment on demand. iPads boast about the speed and ease of downloading information. Because we live in such a fast-paced society, some conclude that spiritual insights should be instantaneous, too. I call this phenomenon fast food spirituality. "Give me a mantra to repeat or a potion to drink," they say, "and I'll get on-the-spot illumination. After all, I'm entitled to it, right?"

> Spirit is an invisible force made visible in all life.
> –Maya Angelou (1928–2014), Singer, writer, activist

Unfortunately, spiritual insights don't happen that way. To attain higher levels of enlightenment, an aspirant should meditate daily, perhaps seek a teacher or study group, exchange ideas with others, read widely on the subject, and most importantly, experience life. After long contemplation of spiritual and philosophical issues, you may be rewarded with some nuggets of perception. Such achievements can take a lifetime to accomplish. In my opinion, the spiritual journey itself represents one of the joys of living on Earth.

At the same time, I believe you can do much to enhance your progress on your chosen path through structured meditations, rhythmic breathing exercises, visualizations, yoga, journaling, and, of course, by creating and consuming potions. These activities help put you in the proper frame of mind to plumb the depths of your subconscious mind and contemplate spiritual topics that resurface in flashes of understanding and wisdom. Following are some potions designed to guide you along the path toward self-realization and enlightenment.

Thoughts on Meditation

Meditation and prayer are important to spiritual development because they help calm the body, balance the personality, and increase self-understanding. When the body is at ease, the mind and spirit will become still, then open like a flower to receive the morning sunshine.

Create a contemplative mood by retiring to somewhere peaceful and quiet. Play soothing background music, light candles, burn your favorite incense. Sometimes a warm bath will help you to ground and center. After that, potions may come into play.

Serves 1

PURIFICATION JUICE

Purify yourself on the inside of your physical body with the following juice. Drink it before engaging in meditation, contemplation, or prayer.

Ingredients

- 1 mango, peeled and seeded
- ½ cup pineapple
- ½ cup pineapple juice
- 1 teaspoon lime juice
- ½ teaspoon cola powder (or ¼ cup cola drink)

Directions

Blend all of the ingredients until smooth and serve in a tall glass.

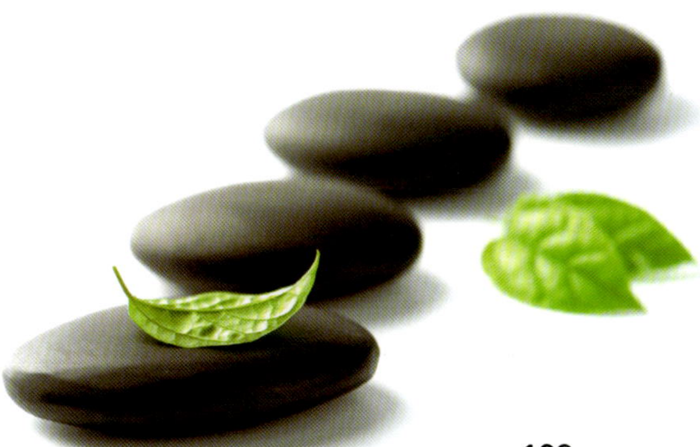

Serves 1

Open My Mind to Higher Powers INFUSION

Perhaps during your next meditation or prayer session you'll wish to seek guidance from Above. To make your mind receptive to direction from a Higher Power, infuse the following tisane.

Ingredients

- 1 cup hot water, filtered
- ½ teaspoon rose hips, crushed
- ¼ teaspoon chamomile flowers
- ¼ teaspoon honeysuckle flowers
- Pinch of powdered clove

Direction

If you can't find the honeysuckle flowers, substitute a splash or two of mango or apple juice.

Serves 1

Someone to Watch Over Me TEA

This lightly infused tea is designed to strengthen the bond between you and your guardian angel or higher self so that you can make contact while sleeping.

Ingredients

- 1 cup hot water
- ½ teaspoon white tea (or 1 white teabag)
- ¼ teaspoon lemon balm, fresh
- ¼ teaspoon cinquefoil, cut and sifted

Directions

Drink it hot at bedtime.

Serves 1

Good Vibrations TEA

To contemplate the nature of happiness and fulfillment, prepare and consume the following infusion.

Ingredients

- 1 cup hot water
- ½ teaspoon loose green tea (or 1 teabag)
- 3 fresh rose petals
- ½ teaspoon dried apple pieces
- ¼ teaspoon blessed thistle, cut and sifted
- ⅛ teaspoon cardamom powder
- Pinch of black pepper

Directions

Boil the water, infuse the ingredients for 2-3 minutes. Serve, and drink while hot.

BOTANICALS WITH SIMILAR PROPERTIES:

Honey
Lemon balm
Motherwort
Pear
Potato

Serves 1

Who Am I and Why Am I Here JUICE?

Contemplate life's mysteries and expand your consciousness with the following juice.

Ingredients

- 1 mango, peeled, seeded, and cut into cubes
- 6 strawberries
- ½ cup organic apple juice
- ¼ teaspoon spikenard
- 3 drops goldenseal extract or pinch of the herb

Directions

Process the mango and strawberries in a blender, add the rest of the ingredients, and blend until well mixed. Blend in 2–3 ice cubes, if desired. Serve in a tall glass.

If you can't find the spikenard or the goldenseal extract, or if for any reason this potion does not appeal, see the Sunday Shake recipe in Chapter 17.

Facilitate Journaling

Some of my friends engaged in expanding their awareness of spiritual topics complain that they have trouble keeping up with their journals. Some can't even decide which of their numerous daily thoughts and experiences to note.

JOURNAL JUICE

Serves 1

If you're having trouble separating the day-to-day from the spiritual, the next potion will help turn your mind inward so you can extract the most worthwhile thoughts to record.

Ingredients

- ½ cup pomegranate juice
- ¼ cup tangerine juice
- ¼ cup peach juice
- ½ teaspoon lemon balm, fresh

Directions

Blend the ingredients together; add ice, if desired. Pour into a glass, and drink. *Bon chance!*

Using the Five Senses to Peer into Other Worlds

Earlier in this book, I talked about the five senses and how you can incorporate them into potion-crafting. When the five senses are engaged by the perfectly balanced interplay of the four elements, your potions are transformed into a symphony of synergy. By this, I mean that the recipes draw on the five senses to help you attain a psychic and spiritual awareness greater than the sum of its parts.

In other words, as a result of drinking your potion, you become imbued with what a layperson might call a sixth sense. This ability may enable you to experience what lies beyond the confines of everyday life. By perceiving something outside our normal realm of experience, if only for a short time, we can harness these perceptions for our own self-improvement as well as to help others. To close this chapter, I wish to share two formulas that have stood me in good stead for this kind of self-development.

To enhance your intuitive perceptions and improve clairvoyance, I recommend mixing a potion according to your personal taste from any of the following ingredients: anise, bay, cinnamon, cinquefoil, cucumber, eyebright, ginger, grape, linden, lovage, marshmallow, meadowsweet, melon (I especially favor honeydew), onion, poppy, rue, sage. Or try the following recipe.

Serves 1

Mind Reader TEA

Photograph by C. Nathan Pulley Photography

Sometimes it is useful to be able to read what's on someone else's mind in order to communicate better with that person. This is especially true if, for example, you happen to be an intuitive reader. Occasionally, the thoughts that the person who has come to you for a reading is unconsciously broadcasting are so intense they can overwhelm your intuitive impressions. This phenomenon tends to occur when the person with whom you wish to communicate is endowed with a strong personality. In such instances, I suggest you prepare the following beverage infusion.

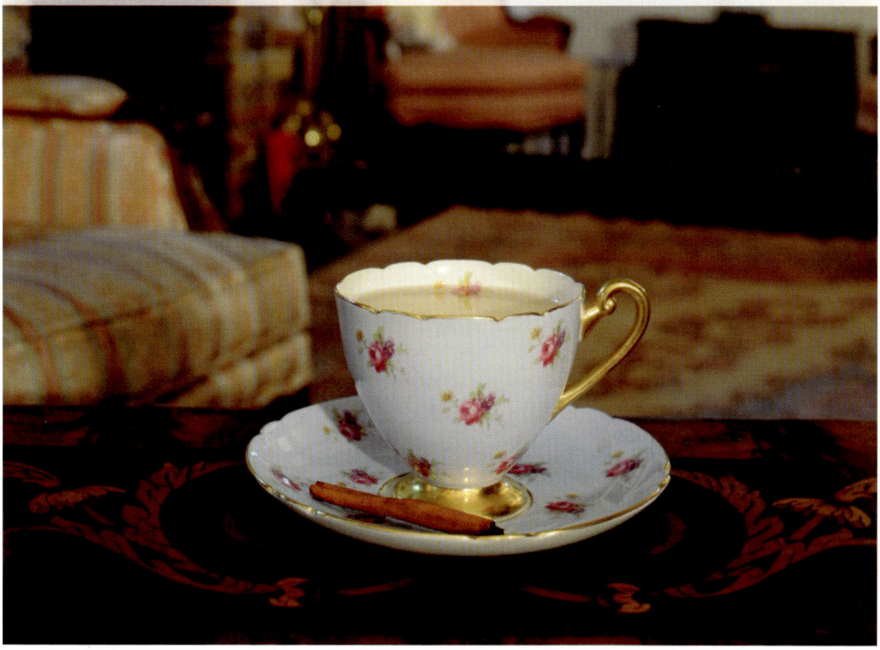

Ingredients

- 1 cup hot water
- ½ teaspoon white tea
- ¼ teaspoon lemon peel
- ¼ teaspoon orange peel
- ¼ teaspoon lavender
- ¼ teaspoon lemon verbena

Directions

Do not sweeten this brew, as sweet and milky substances tend to dilute some people's intuitive abilities. It's sweet enough anyway with the citrus peels. Before drinking, stir the tea with a cinnamon stick. You can also rub a few drops of this tisane on your temples and third eye—the space between your eyebrows. Also known as the *ajna* brow chakra in some Eastern religions, it is thought to lead to inner realms of higher consciousness. And remember to use this potion in an ethical way.

Serves 1

What Will the Future Bring? INFUSION

Hawaiians have enjoyed kava-kava as an intuition enhancer for centuries. If taken before retiring, it is alleged to confer epic length, prophetic dreams.

Ingredients	Directions
1 cup hot water ½ teaspoon kava-kava root ½ teaspoon lemon balm ¼ teaspoon meadowsweet	Infuse the ingredients in the hot water. Serve and drink before retiring.

COLA DRINKS AND COLA NUT

Cucumber	Parsley
Melon	Sweet peppers

I hope that the future you see for yourself is filled with blessings and joy and that it will create beautiful memories. To help ensure that your journey on the road to happiness is safe and smooth, the next chapter will undertake potions for security and protection.

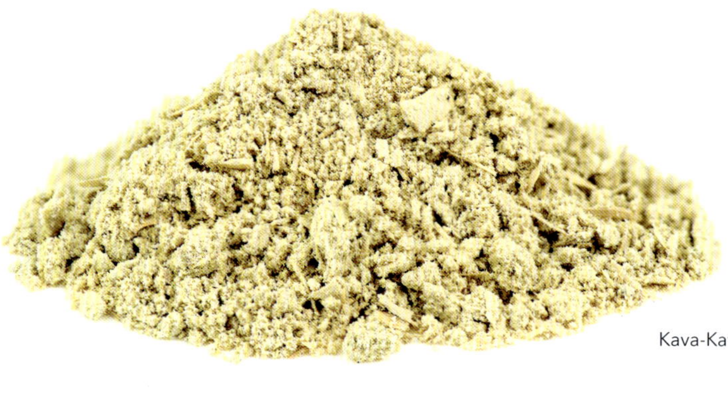

Kava-Kava Root

Chapter 16

SAFE HARBORS

Potions for Safety and Protection

Physical safety and protection have been a concern from time immemorial, and contemporary times are no different. Mental and emotional security are equally important. In this chapter I have selected formulas to cover a range of situations.

Some people occasionally become fixated with the notion that they need strong protection from enemies hell-bent on ruining their lives. Sometimes the threat is very real, yet the danger can also emanate from the individual's own psyche. A person can turn the perceived threat into a self-fulfilling prophecy simply by dwelling on negative thoughts. Think of this as the reverse of Norman Vincent Peale's famous power of positive thinking. By creating negative thought forms, you may plunge into a downward spiral, which if not caught in time can wreak irreversible effects.

To banish negative thoughts, I recommend that you meditate on the problem. Petition for guidance from whatever deity you conceive of as the All-One and drink the following juice.

Serves 1

Banish Negative Thoughts JUICE

This potion contains a small amount of the bitter herb, hyssop, which has been used for purification since ancient times by the Hebrews and other cultures.

Ingredients

- 2 tablespoons white grape juice
- ¾ cup red grape juice
- 1 teaspoon fresh lemon balm leaves, chopped (or dried, if it's winter and you can't find it fresh)
- 1 teaspoon honey
- ¼ teaspoon hyssop, cut and sifted

Directions

If desired, put a little fizz into the potion by adding carbonated water to taste. Stir with a spoon, and drink.

Serves 1-2

Black Belt of Protection SMOOTHIE

Photograph by C. Nathan Pulley Photography

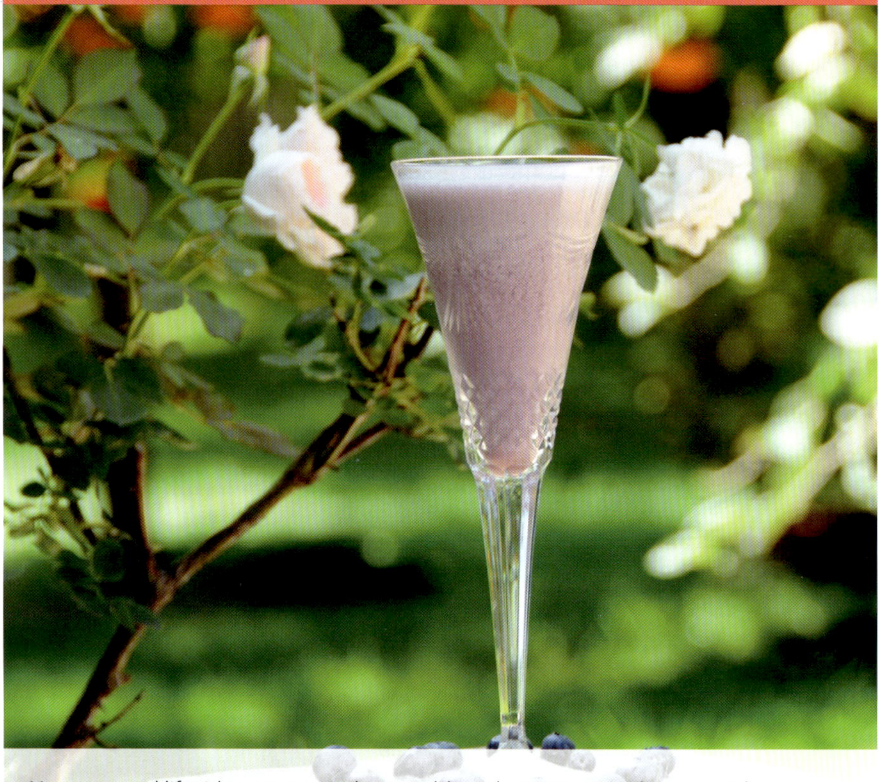

Your personal life tide seems at its lowest ebb and everyone you know is picking some nit with you. Fortify yourself with the following smoothie. It will help erect an invisible shield around you to discourage any negative vibes aimed your way.

Ingredients

- ½ cup blueberry juice
- 1 tablespoon Earl Grey tea, steeped for 5 minutes, cooled
- ½ cup coconut water
- 1 cup coconut ice cream or frozen yogurt

Directions

Blend the ingredients and pour into a shake glass. Drink before heading out for the day.

OTHER BOTANICALS WITH SIMILAR ALLEGED PROPERTIES:

Cinquefoil
Red clover blossom
Cranberry juice (for mental and emotional self-defense)
Garlic
Grapefruit juice (for physical protection)
Solomon's seal
Tomato

Serves 1-2

Defend Against Nightmares SMOOTHIE

Whether your nightmares originate in the ill will of others or your own fears, this bedtime smoothie will help relax and protect you. Liquefy it in a blender.

Ingredients

- 1 mango, peeled, pitted, and cut into cubes
- ½ cup fresh pineapple, cubed
- 2 tablespoons canned pumpkin
- ½ teaspoon cinnamon
- ¼ teaspoon clove
- 1 cup vanilla ice cream or low fat frozen yogurt

Directions

Blend together the first five ingredients; add the frozen dessert, and blend again until smooth.

OTHER BOTANICALS REPUTED TO BANISH NEGATIVITY AND VILLAINS FROM YOUR ENVIRONMENT:

Agrimony
Almond
Basil
Bergamot
Calendula (allegedly helps identify robbers)
Cayenne
Clove
White clover
Flax
Gentian
Grape
Horehound
Valerian

Serves 1

Banish Nightmares for Your Child COCOA

The prior potion works for both adults and children, but if you want to try something different for your kids, treat them to a bedtime cup of hot cocoa.

Ingredients

- Unsweetened cocoa prepared according to directions
- Sweetener, to taste
- Marshmallows
- Caraway seeds, crushed

Directions

Prepare this recipe from unsweetened cocoa and add sweetener to taste. I suggest you go light on the sugar, as it can lead to hyperactivity. Not what you want to achieve at bedtime. Top with marshmallows instead of whipped cream. If they don't mind the taste, add a couple of crushed caraway seeds to the brew. They should sleep like angels with no fear of the monster hiding under the bed.

Although this is a book about drinkable potions, not aromatherapy, I'd like to add one aromatherapeutic tip for your child's bedroom. Lime essence in an aroma diffuser works wonders to relax your little one before bedtime.

Serves 2

Make Friends of Your Enemy TEA

There comes a time, it is hoped, when you desire and are in a position to offer the peace pipe–in this case, a peace potion–to an enemy. Bury the hatchet by inviting your former nemesis to share a cup of the following tea.

Ingredients

- 2 cups hot water
- 1 teaspoon Earl Grey tea
- ¼ teaspoon fresh basil
- Lemon slices for garnish

Directions

I usually recommend taking tea without a sweetener. In this potion a teaspoon of honey or sugar will metaphorically help the medicine go down—at least according to Mary Poppins. Prepare and garnish with a slices of lemon before drinking. To the good health and welfare of you both!

Serves as many as prepared

Discourage Unwanted Visitors INFUSION

Have you ever wished those party animal friends of yours would just quit and go home? Besides removing the liquor, which can put an instantaneous damper on any party, try offering your guests a final cup of cheer.

Ingredients

- Hot water, 1 cup for each guest
- Blueberry teabag, 1 for each guest
- Pinch or two of spearmint, per cup

Directions

Prepare a beverage infusion from the blueberry teabags and add the spearmint as a garnish.

Serves 4-6

Family Comfort
LEEK AND POTATO SOUP

To calm your family and keep loved ones from harm during any crisis, serve this soup at lunch or dinnertime.

Ingredients

- 2 tablespoons butter
- 1 leek, cleaned, peeled, and chopped
- 4 cups water
- 1–2 chicken bouillon cubes
- Salt and pepper to taste
- 2 potatoes, peeled and diced
- 1 carrot, diced
- 2–4 cups milk
- 2 tablespoons bacon, crumbled (or "faux" bacon bits made from soy)
- 1 tablespoon fresh parsley, chopped

Directions

Melt the butter and cook the chopped leek in it until tender. Add the water, bouillon cube(s), and salt and pepper, and bring to a boil. Add the potatoes and carrots and cook until the liquid is reduced to 2 cups. Cool; then put the mixture through a blender. Return it to the pot and add enough milk to make a soupy consistency. Bring the soup to a boil again and simmer for 10 minutes. Serve in bowls and sprinkle with bacon bits or soy bacon and fresh chopped parsley.

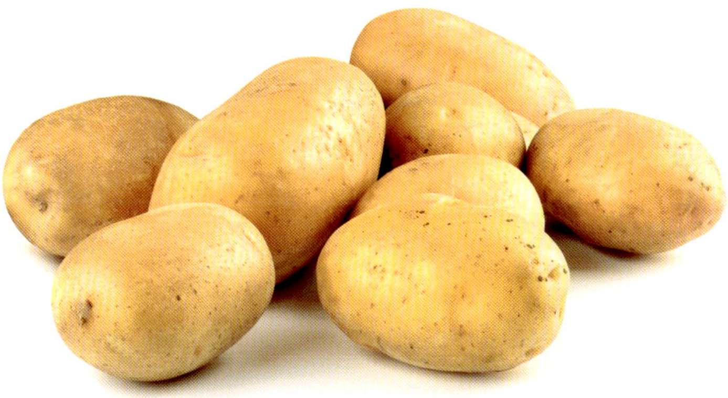

Chapter 17

POTIONS FOR ALL OCCASIONS

As we come to the end of this part of the book, I'd like to share a few recipes for celebratory occasions, beginning with the days of the week. They represent a fine reason to drink a healthy potion—as if you needed an excuse! Sometimes I list a specific botanical with more than one day. This is because different esoteric and ancient traditions sometimes disagree on the associations.

Days of the Week Potions

Serves 1-2

Monday
AGUA DE MELÓN (Cantaloupe Water)

Here's another Mexican *agua fresca* treat from Shauna Sanstead-Corona.

Ingredients

- 1 cantaloupe
- 4 cups water
- Organic sugar, sweeten to taste

Directions

Take 1 cantaloupe: grind the flesh, pulp and seeds with water in a blender, and strain. Add as much pulp as you want to the water and sweeten to taste with organic sugar.

OTHER BOTANICALS ASSOCIATED WITH THIS DAY:

Banana
Cabbage
Cauliflower
Cucumber
Dulse (a kind of seaweed)
Lotus root
Marshmallow
Mushroom
Papaya
Potato
Turnip
Leafy vegetables

Serves 4

Tuesday PUNCH

This potion is sure to fortify you to tackle any challenge or project that may gallop your way

Ingredients

- 3 cups water
- 1 6-oz. can cranberry concentrate, frozen
- 3 tablespoons honey
- 6 cinnamon sticks, broken in pieces
- 6 whole cloves
- 1 teaspoon cardamom, ground
- 1 cup red grape juice

Directions

Heat the water, cranberry juice concentrate, honey, cinnamon, cloves, cardamom, and red grape juice to a boil. Reduce heat; cover, and simmer for 10 minutes. Strain out the spices. If you are making the brew alcoholic, stir in the wine and *crème de cassis* now. Heat thoroughly again, but do not boil. Serve in mugs. Garnish with a cinnamon stick, if desired.

*If you wish to make this brew alcoholic, substitute 2 cups of dry red wine and ½ cup *crème de cassis* for 2 cups of the water.

OTHER BOTANICALS ASSOCIATED WITH THIS DAY:

Allspice
Basil
Caper
Chive
Coffee (although some link coffee with Sunday)
Coriander
Galangal
Garlic
Ginger
Hops
Horseradish
Mustard
Nettle
Onion
Parsley
Pepper
Radish
Sarsaparilla

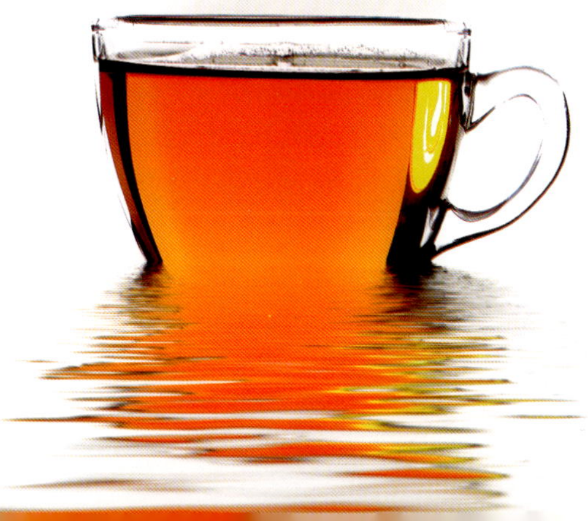

Serves a crowd

Wednesday

ORANGE BLOSSOM PUNCH

What better way to celebrate midweek than to prepare and serve this tasty punch? Many of the ingredients in this recipe are not traditionally associated with this day, but the orange color of the punch is. Wednesday belongs to Mercury, the swift-footed god of myth. In various traditions, Mercury participates in the affairs of all the deities, hence, all the days of the week, and by analogy, all ingredients.

Ingredients

- 2 6-ounce cans frozen pineapple juice, thawed
- 2 6-ounce cans orange juice concentrate, thawed
- 3 liters chilled spritzer water
- 1 cup orange slices
- 1 cup cranberry slices

Directions

Stir together all of the ingredients. Pour over ice and stir well again.

This punch can also be served on occasions when you wish to draw together a group of like-minded people, as described in Chapter 14. The potion is designed to encourage those interested in becoming contributing members of the group to come together and work in harmony.

* If you prefer an alcoholic refreshment, add ⍰ cup of Grand Marnier and substitute champagne for the spritzer water.

OTHER BOTANICALS ASSOCIATED WITH THIS DAY

Anise
Brazil nut
Caraway, carrots
Celery
Cinnamon
Dill
Filbert
Hazelnut
Horehound
Lavender
Lemon
Licorice
Bee balm
Oat
Orange blossom
Parsley
Parsnip
Pomegranate
Tangerine
Valerian
Lemon verbena

Serves 2

Thursday

APRICOT-FIG EGGNOG

This recipe is an updated version of an ancient formula to honor Jupiter and Thor, mythical lords of this day.

Ingredients

- 2 eggs
- 2 tablespoons honey
- 1 cup apricot nectar
- 4 figs, seeded
- ¾ cup orange juice
- ½ cup nonfat dry milk powder
- 2 tablespoons protein powder
- 1 tablespoon lemon juice
- 1 cup frozen strawberries, partially thawed
- Fresh mint leaf, strawberry slice, or lemon peel curl for garnish

Directions

In a small mixer, beat the eggs until thick and lemon-colored. Gradually add the honey, beating constantly. Set aside. In a blender, combine the apricot nectar, figs, orange juice, milk powder, protein powder, and lemon juice. Cover and blend until well mixed. Add the strawberries; blend again until smooth.

With the blender running at low speed, add the egg mixture. Blend again until smooth. Transfer the mixture to a storage container; cover and chill. Stir well before serving. Garnish each serving with a fresh mint leaf, strawberry slice, or lemon peel curl.

OTHER BOTANICALS ASSOCIATED WITH THIS DAY:

Asparagus
Borage
Carnation (yes, the flowers are edible, but they don't blend well in liquid potions–use them instead as a garnish)
Chestnut
Clove
Clover
Dandelion
Endive
Jasmine flower
Lemon balm
Maple syrup
Nutmeg
Rose hip
Saffron
Star anise
Sugar

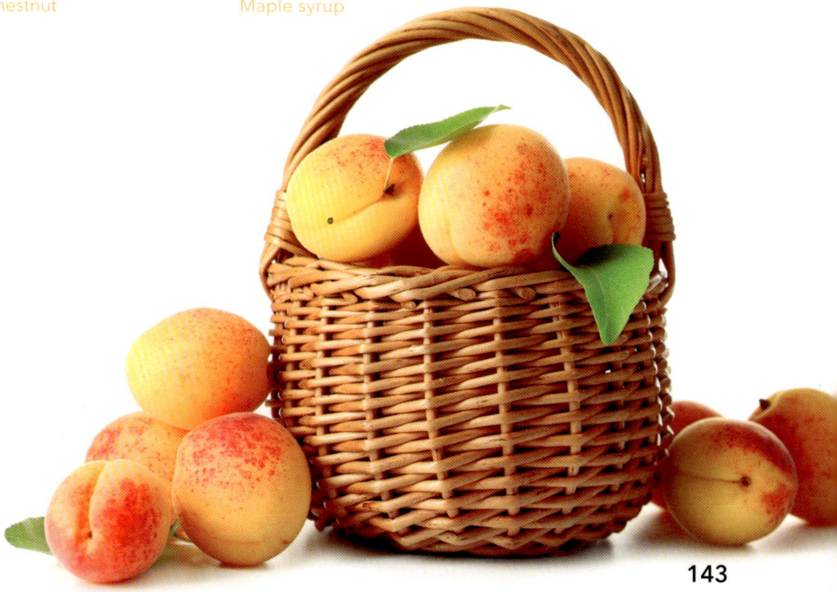

Serves 1 (multiply the recipe for each additional guest)

Friday
MILK PUNCH

Here's a potion guaranteed to spark your weekend. It contains alcohol, which can be left out. A reasonable substitute for the whiskey is non-alcoholic buttered rum extract, available through Frontier Products Cooperative and elsewhere. You can also substitute a shot glass of milk.

Ingredients

- 1 egg
- 1 teaspoon sugar
- Dash of salt
- Dash of vanilla extract
- 1 shot of whiskey, if desired
- ½ teaspoon cardamom seeds

Directions

Beat the ingredients together. Pour into a punch glass and sprinkle with nutmeg.

OTHER BOTANICALS ASSOCIATED WITH THIS DAY

Almond
Aloe vera
Apple
Apricot
Avocado
Banana
Bean
Blackberry
Cardamom
Caraway
Cherry
Coriander
Elderberry
Gooseberry
Honeysuckle
Huckleberry
Passion flower
Peach
Pear
Plantain
Raspberry
Rose
Thyme
Vanilla
Vervain

Serves 4

Saturday
TAMARIND FRUIT WATER

Make this Mexican sweetened water in much the same way as indicated for the *agua de jamaica* water from Chapter 1.

Ingredients

- 1 tamarind
- 1 quart water
- ⅛ cup sugar (or other sweetner), to taste

Directions

To prepare the tamarind, remove the shell, put the seeds in a quart of water, and boil for 15 minutes or until the pulp loosens. When this mixture cools, loosen all the pulp from the seeds with your fingers. Remove any stringy matter that may stick to the pulp. Add a cup of the pulp to a quart of water and about ⅛ cup of sugar, or other sweetener to taste. Stir well and serve.

OTHER BOTANICALS ASSOCIATED WITH THIS DAY:

Barley
Beechnut
Beet
Juniper
Pomegranate
Quince

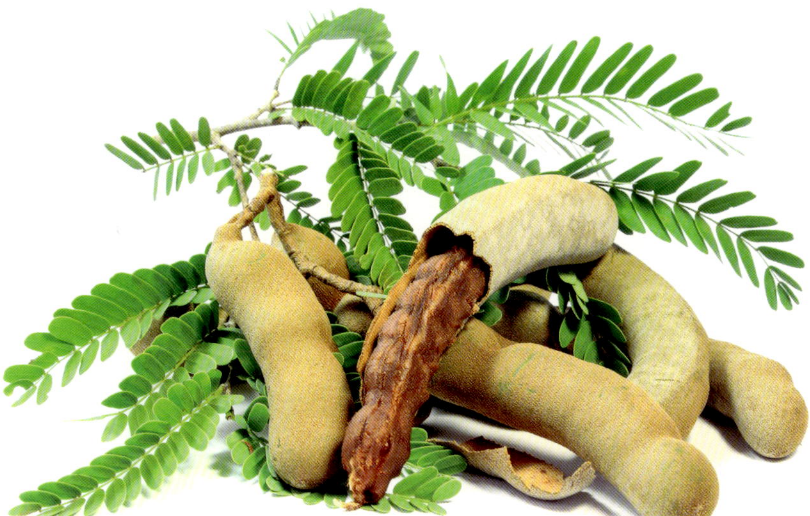

Serves 2 (or more)

Sunday SHAKE

Who am I really? What is my purpose in life? Here is a formula to sip on a lazy Sunday afternoon when things have quieted down around your house. It will help enhance your meditations on this heady topic.

Ingredients

- ½ pint coconut ice cream
- 1 cup (8 ounces) canned, crushed pineapple
- ¾ cup light cream
- 3 ounces frozen tangerine juice (½ of a 6-ounce can. Save the rest to make a juice to add a little gusto to your life.)
- 1 small banana
- ½ cup ice cubes
- ¼ cup shredded coconut
- Rose petals or shredded coconut for garnish, if desired

Directions

Blend all of the ingredients until smooth. If you wish, garnish with toasted, shredded coconut and a fresh rose petal or two.

OTHER BOTANICALS ASSOCIATED WITH THIS DAY

Almond
Bayberry
Cashew
Chicory
Cinnamon
Citrus fruit
Chamomile
Galangal
Ginseng
Honey
Pineapple
Saffron
Sesame
Tea
Vanilla
Walnut

Seasonal Potions

Here are several potion recipes to ring in any season of the year. As an aside, many old books of food traditions and lore list onion as an appropriate botanical to celebrate any season.

Serves 4

New Year PEA SOUP

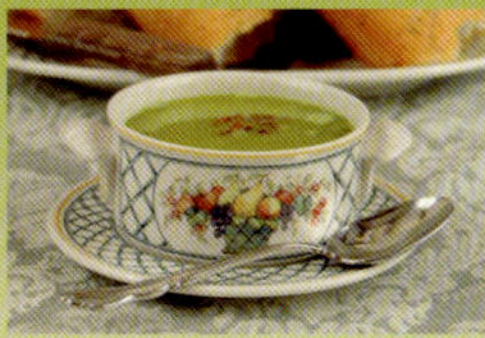

An old superstition states that if you eat peas on New Year's Day, you will prosper throughout the entire year. Other traditions claim that eating peas will keep you motivated and give you direction. Need I add that peas are a super food rich in vitamins and minerals that will help guard your health throughout the winter months? The following easy-to-prepare recipe, a family favorite in our household, makes a delicious way to celebrate anticipated joys to come. Although it calls for fresh peas, I have found frozen peas to be equally sweet.

Ingredients

- 1 cup peas, fresh or frozen
- 3 tablespoons butter, cubed
- 2 teaspoons flour
- ½ teaspoon ginger
- 3 cups chicken broth (or 3 cups water and 3 teaspoons chicken broth granules)
- Salt and pepper, to taste
- Bacon bits or soy bacon to garnish, if desired

Directions

Blend all of the ingredients thoroughly in a food processor. Don't worry that the butter and flour may look somewhat lumpy; they will soon smooth out. After blending, transfer the mixture to a saucepan and heat to boiling, stirring constantly. Boil for 3-4 minutes. Stir in salt and pepper to taste, and serve. Garnish with bacon bits or soy bacon, if desired.

Serves 6 or more

Winter WASSAIL BOWL

Celebrate the shortest day of the year and the beginning of the waxing year, along with its promise of renewed energy, life, and hope with the following punch.

Ingredients

- 1 cup water
- ½ teaspoon nutmeg
- 1 ginger root, bruised (or ¼ teaspoon powdered ginger)
- 1 cinnamon stick
- 1 teaspoon cloves, whole
- 1 teaspoon allspice berries, whole
- 4-6 apples, roasted and sliced (optional)
- ¼ teaspoon coriander seeds
- ¼ teaspoon cardamom seeds
- 1 quart ginger ale
- 6 egg yolks, beaten until lemony-looking
- 6 egg whites, beaten until frothy
- Sugar to taste

Directions

Boil the water in a pot. Add the spices; reduce the heat and simmer for 10 minutes. Remove the pot from the heat. Then add the ginger ale. Slowly beat in the yolks and whites separately, beating constantly. The punch is ready to serve in mugs. Garnish with the apple slices if you are serving the punch in a bowl.

* If you'd like an alcoholic potion, supplement this brew with ½ bottle of sherry, in which case you may want to increase the sugar to 2 cups.

Serves 2

First Light of Spring SMOOTHIE

Welcome in the spring with this smoothie

Ingredients

- ½ cup blackberries (Fresh is nice, but given the fact that blackberries are often out of season in most places, frozen berries will do.)
- ½ cup fresh pineapple, peeled and chopped
- 1 tablespoon heather honey (I admit I'm spoiled from living in the UK, where heather honey is readily available. You can substitute clover honey.)
- 1 pint frozen vanilla yogurt

Directions

Blend the berries and pineapple for 30 seconds. Add the frozen yogurt and honey, and blend until smooth.

A simpler variation on this recipe is a juice that calls for blackberry juice steeped with a few rose hips and a couple of drops of vanilla extract.

Serves a crowd

Summer PUNCH

Six months ago, you rang in the New Year and the shortest day with a winter wassail bowl. So it makes sense to celebrate high summer with this refreshing punch.

Ingredients

- 4 oranges, unpeeled
- 6 cups fresh, squeezed orange juice
- 1 bottle carbonated water (1 liter)
- Juice of 1 lemon
- Sweetener of your choice to taste
- Block of ice
- 4 dashes of aromatic bitters, if desired
- Small bottle of maraschino cherries for garnish
- Apple slices for garnish

Directions

Slice the oranges into 1-inch cartwheels, cut the cartwheels in half. If desired, place the oranges in a shallow glass dish and pour 1 pint of brandy over the oranges. Chill overnight. Chill all of the other ingredients, too. Before serving, combine the water, lemon, juices, and sugar. Stir the sugar to dissolve it, and pour the entire mixture over a block of ice in a large punch bowl. Add the orange slices, and, if marinated in brandy, the brandy as well. Stir slightly to mix. Garnish with cherries and apple slices.

Serves 1-2

Dog Days of August LEMON COOLER

At this time of year in days of old, villagers gathered to sell livestock and garden produce and partake in games of strength, dancing, and general celebration. You may simply want to celebrate this time of year by settling back in a recliner in the shade and sipping this refreshing drink.

Ingredients

- 1 cup ice cold water
- ¼ cup lemon juice
- ¼ can frozen lemonade
- ¼ cup organic sugar
- 1 large serving vanilla ice cream
- ½ teaspoon cardamom, ground
- 1 teaspoon borage tops, chopped

Directions

Place all of the ingredients in a blender, cover, and process until smooth. Your cooler is ready to drink.

Serves a crowd

HALLOWEEN BREW

Honor this final harvest time of year (as well as all of those little trick-or-treaters) with the following cider.

Ingredients

- 1 gallon apple cider
- 6 cinnamon sticks
- 1 teaspoon cloves, whole
- 1 teaspoon allspice, whole
- 1 tablespoon hot cinnamon candies
- Apple slices for garnish

Directions

Combine the ingredients in a large cauldron or pot; simmer gently for 30 minutes. Garnish with fresh apple slices. Serve hot.

Serves a crowd

Celebration Kir CHAMPAGNE PUNCH

Photograph by C. Nathan Pulley Photography

My final recipe is unabashedly alcoholic as I've never found a non-alcoholic substitute that can replicate the taste. Celebrate any occasion with the following punch.

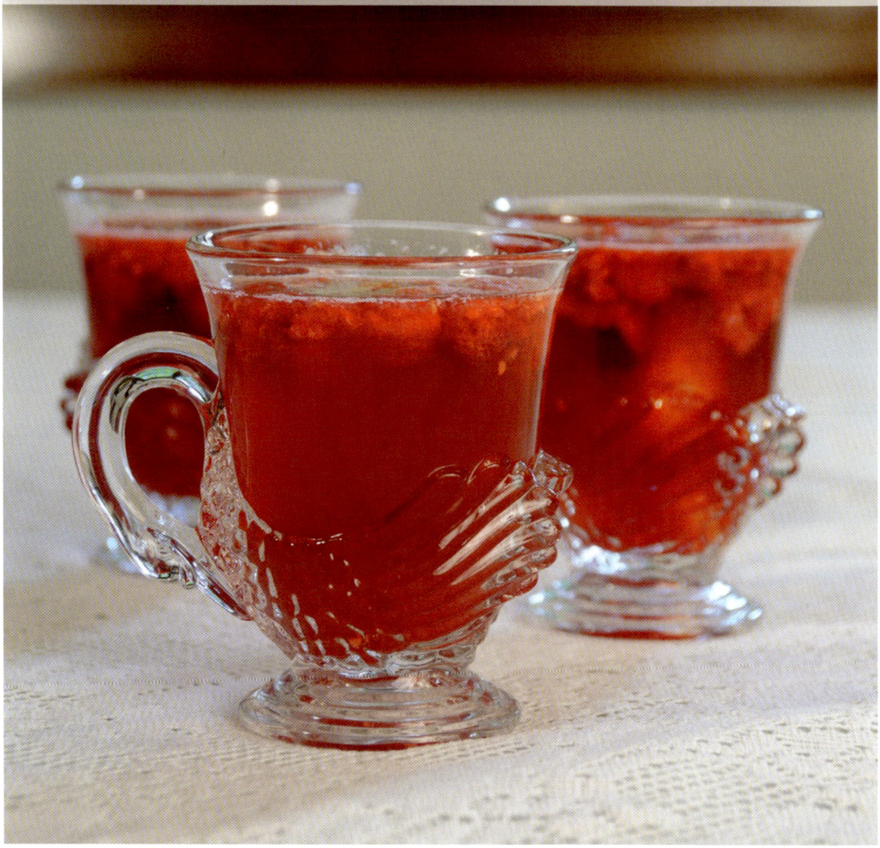

Ingredients

- 1 package frozen raspberries, pureed
- 1 can mandarin oranges
- 2 10-ounce packages frozen raspberries, partially thawed
- 32 ounces sparkling water, chilled
- 1 cup *crème de cassis*, chilled
- 3 bottles champagne, chilled

Directions

In advance, pour the pureed raspberries into a ring mold. Add the can of mandarin oranges, stir well, and freeze.

Before the party, combine the rest of the ingredients in a punch bowl and stir well. Take the mold from the freezer, remove it from the ring, and place it on top of the punch.

Serves about 4 (depending on the size of the glasses)

Thanksgiving for the Harvest SMOOTHIE

Save this smoothie for a healthy Thanksgiving treat. It tastes like liquid pumpkin pie. Pumpkin is a signature vegetable of the season.

Ingredients

- 1 cup low fat milk
- 2 tablespoons honey
- 1 cup solid-packed pumpkin
- 1 cup banana, sliced
- 2 cups vanilla low fat frozen yogurt
- 2 tablespoons dark brown organic sugar
- 1 teaspoon cinnamon
- ½ teaspoon allspice powder
- ½ teaspoon powdered ginger
- ¼ teaspoon clove powder

Directions

Mix all of the ingredients in a blender on low speed until combined. Continue mixing gradually, increasing the speed until smooth. Pour into glasses and garnish with dried apple slices dusted in cinnamon on a cinnamon stick.

General Potion Strengtheners

If you desire a particularly potent potion, add small amounts of any of the following ingredients: cinnamon, couch grass, damiana, ginseng extract, guaraná seeds, lemon, protein powder, rosemary, saffron. When you need a potion to take effect immediately, add a couple of drops of any of these extracts: almond, ginger, peppermint.

I hope these recipes, as well as the other information I have provided in this book, have kept you healthy and helped you achieve your heart's desire. Although there are still the appendices, glossary, and bibliography to browse at your leisure, I leave you now with this Irish blessing:

Part III

APPENDIX A

Fruits and Vegetables

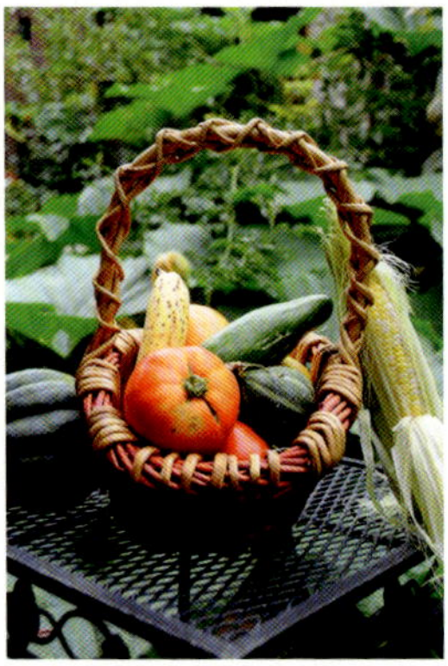

Harvest Basket of Fruits and Vegetables.

This appendix describes common fruits and vegetables for potion-crafting. So you can easily identify the plant, the first thing you will see listed under an entry is the scientific designation. I go on to describe the plant, give culinary uses, and indicate some of the botanical's nutritional benefits. Finally, I spin tales of some of the plant's lore to fire your imagination to create super potions that will knock people's socks off. This information, together with the formulas from Part II, should provide you with a fairly comprehensive guide to personalize your recipes.

Throughout this appendix, especially in the sections dedicated to lore, you will find references to planets, zodiac signs, and deities from mythology and folklore. Long ago, our forefathers developed a theory that conceived of plants as part of the interconnected system of the cosmos. They named their theory the Doctrine of Signatures. This theory posits that everything in the universe is in some way linked to something else. Think of it as a sort of pre-scientific, intuitive quantum physics.

According to this doctrine, plants show their associations by manifesting a recognizable form, color, scent, habitat, and connection to a heavenly body, which in turn links to a deity or several deities from mythology. Sometimes these associations connect in some observable way to the human body. For example, the seaweed bladderwrack is composed of little sacks that resemble miniature human bladders. This plant was prescribed to cure urinary tract infections long before scientific studies corroborated its diuretic effects. The red color of pomegranate juice closely resembles human blood, so this fruit was given to patients to help cure blood and heart disorders. Modern science has since found that pomegranates support the heart and blood circulation. Coincidence? Perhaps. At any rate, I include these associations because they can help you decide which fruits and vegetables to use in your formulas from a psychological perspective.

I also offer folkloric meanings from a compendium of floral knowledge known as *The Language of Flowers*. Since smelling food is a big part of tasting it, scent plays an important psychological role in the culinary arts, including potion-crafting. The *Language of Flowers* originated in a French book written in 1840 by Madame de la Tour, who researched the symbolic meanings for plants from folklore, mythology, art, and literature. She also incorporated an eighteenth-century work by Lady Mary Wortley Montagu, wife of the British Ambassador to a Turkish sultan. Lady Montagu developed a list of Eastern connotations for plants and flowers that she compiled from interviews with her Asian friends.

Here are the ingredients. I hope you let your imagination run wild with them and that you find concocting your individualized potions fulfilling and enjoyable.

ALMOND

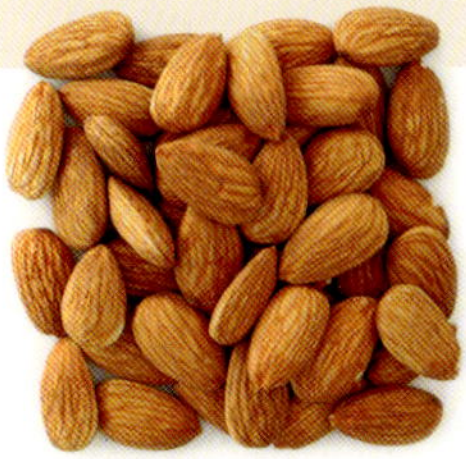

(Prunus amygdalus communis)

Description: The tasty nuts of this pink-flowering tree and the extract derived from them are the part of the tree used for crafting potions. You may recognize the fruity scent of the flower as the hallmark of Jergen's Lotion.

Culinary Uses: Almond extract lends the characteristic fruity flavor to Mexican hot chocolate that sets it apart from other similar drinks. Sweet almonds can also be simmered in milk and the broth added to soups and sauces to make them more full-bodied.

Lately, almond milk has been touted as a non-lactose alternative to cow's milk. It is readily available at the supermarket, but for those interested in creating their own almond milk potion, here is a recipe.

ALMOND MILK

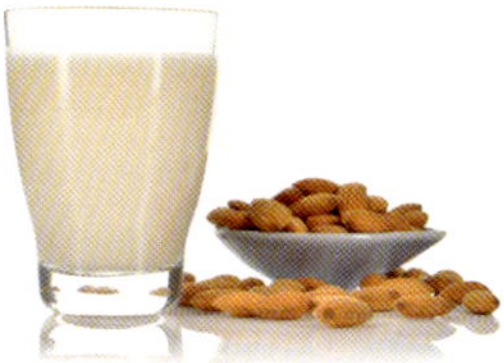

SERVES AROUND 4

Ingredients

- 1 cup whole almonds or almond slivers, blanched to remove skins
- 3 cups spring water
- 1 teaspoon honey

Directions: Combine all of the ingredients in a blender, cover, and process at low speed for 1 minute. Switch to high speed and blend until smooth. Strain the mixture through a cheese cloth to remove any leftover solids. Refrigerate until ready to use. Like cow's milk, almond milk provides a base for smoothies.

Nutrition: In the Middle Ages, pilgrims traveled with almonds in their pockets because they believed that the nuts would sustain them if they had to go without food or water. They also thought that the nut extract cured drunkenness. The pilgrims may have been wrong about the alcoholism cure, but it turns out that almonds are quite nutritious. They are low in cholesterol and sodium and brim with vitamins such as E and D and minerals like manganese, magnesium, potassium, calcium, and iron. The nut contains high amounts of heart-healthy mono-saturated fat, too. Snacking on them helps reduce LDL cholesterol. Odorless, sweet almond oil makes a fine emollient and luxuriant massage oil.

Lore: According to Greek legend, Phyllis killed herself when she thought her lover had deserted her. The gods changed her into a beautiful flowering almond tree. Ever since, the almond has been a symbol of undying love; consequently it is associated with Venus and love. Strangely, in the *Language of Flowers* almond means "stupidity," "indiscretion," and "thoughtlessness," probably because of Phyllis' impetuous act. Almonds also were sacred to the deities Artemis (Greek) and Ptah (Egyptian).

In the Brazilian pantheon, the tree is linked to the sun god, the creator god, and the souls of the dead. Adherents of Brazilian mystery religions believe that the oil carries away the so-called negative fluids or vibrations that accumulate in the temple during the day and releases them into the air far away at night.

Add almond extract to potions to improve business and fertility and to gain wisdom.

APPLE

(Malus genus, Pyrus malus)

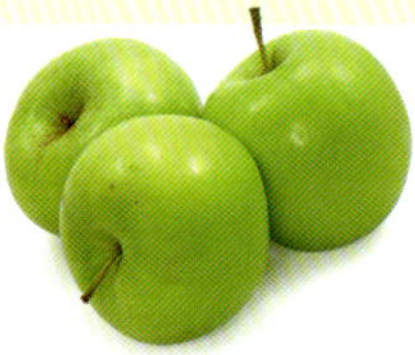

Description: The apple's reputation as the forbidden fruit of the Garden of Eden indicates how long this tree has been around. It is thought to have originated in Central Asia, but the Greeks, as far as anyone knows, were the first to cultivate the tree in orchards.

Over 1,400 varieties are grown worldwide, including eaters, cookers, crab, and cider apples. Popular varieties include granny smith, McIntosh, red and golden delicious, jonagold, and Fuji. Always choose apples that emit a sweet-smelling aroma. If non-organic, or waxed, peel away the skin before juicing.

Culinary Uses: Because apples aid digestion, they are served with fatty meats like goose and pork. Drink apple juice with this type of meal to produce the same effect. Core your apples before juicing or cooking, or buy organic juice at the grocery.

Nutrition: Undoubtedly you've heard the old saw, "An apple a day keeps the doctor away." Indeed, apples are a nutritious fruit. They are loaded with the fiber pectin, which traps cholesterol and whisks it out of the bloodstream. They also contain niacin, magnesium, and vitamin K for the heart. The folic acid content is important to women's health. Vitamins A, B, and C fight stress and promote immunity against disease. Calcium makes for strong bones, and the choloragenic acid is a potential cancer fighter.

Lore: The apple was one of the trees sacred to the Druids of the British Isles. They beheld in this fruit a symbol of immortality, wisdom, and poetry. And so, they named their sacred island Avalon, the "Isle of the Apple Trees" (reputed to be modern-day Glastonbury, England).

Apples comprise an important element of fertility potions and formulas to contact one's guardian angel or higher self as well as to gain wisdom, peace, happiness, and a tranquil ambience in the home. In the *Language of Flowers,* apple blossoms stand for "preference." Since the blossom is both a fruit and flower, supposedly it is favored.

APRICOT

(Prunus armeniaca)

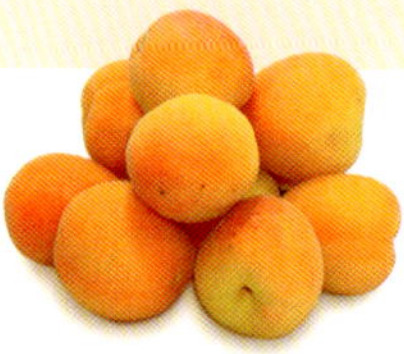

Description: This small, extremely sweet orange-colored fruit of a tree native to Central Asia has been cultivated since approximately 2200 BCE. Apricots hail from the same family as peaches. Select only those fruits that are firm (not mushy) and orange-colored. Green or yellow fruits may be under-ripe.

Culinary Uses: Remove the stone before juicing. Besides making fantastic smoothies, jams, and desserts, apricots comprise an interesting ingredient in chicken, turkey, and game stuffing.

Nutrition: In cultures where people are blessed with long life spans, they often attribute their longevity to a diet rich in this fruit. Apricots contain iron, copper, and some cobalt, so they make an excellent natural supplement for anemia. The high beta-carotene content also fights off cancer. Two bits of advice:

Apricots are a natural laxative (which I found out when I overindulged in the bumper crop from the tree in my garden).

They contain up to six times the sugar as other fresh fruit; so diabetics beware!

Lore: Rumor has it that the apricot was the real apple in the Garden of Eden. Use them in beauty potions, including those taken internally, and in facials. They are also an ingredient of love potions.

ARTICHOKE

(Cynara scolymus)

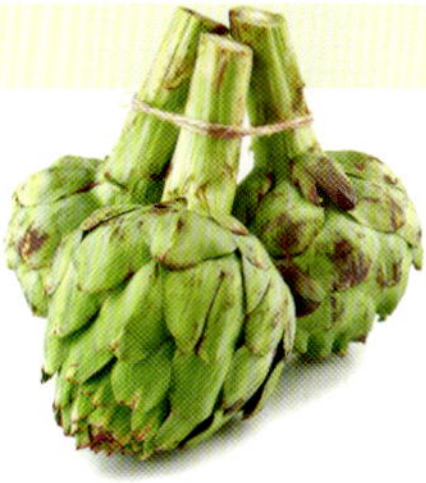

Description: Artichokes look like tiny cabbages, only with smaller, thicker leaves that end in spiky points. They open like a flower when boiled.

Culinary Uses: The nutty-flavored globes are boiled whole. Only eat the soft parts of the leaves and the heart. Marinated artichoke hearts add pizzazz to pizza and pasta. Save the water in which the artichoke was boiled and use as a vegetable soup base.

Nutrition: Artichokes contain compounds similar to caffeine that help you remain alert. Some of the acids found in artichoke hearts activate the liver. The cynarin content helps keep serum triglyceride levels low.

Lore: The famous seventeenth-century herbalist Culpeper linked the artichoke with the planet Venus and the goddess Aphrodite, so today it is an ingredient of love spells. Perhaps because of the prickly leaf tops, artichokes are also added to potions for personal safety and protection.

ASPARAGUS

(Asparagus officinalis)

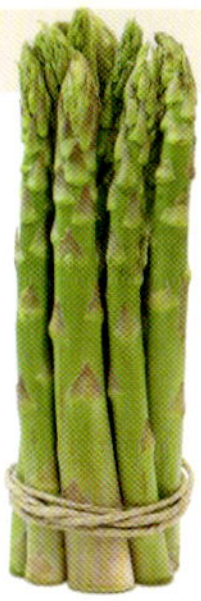

Description: This Mediterranean native of the lily family has been cultivated for over 2,000 years. From early spring until July, the plant sends up tender, green, tightly budded white or purple spears. The shoots carpet the steppes of Russia and some parts of England where cattle and horses graze. If you let asparagus grow, it transforms into a willowy five-foot fern. When buying asparagus, choose bunches that are straight with closed tops, for they are freshest. In the early spring, select thinner stalks, but as the growing season progresses, go for thicker ones. When you get home, slice the stems at the bottom to get a fresh cut, wrap them in paper towels, and store in the coldest part of the refrigerator.

Culinary Uses: Asparagus has been eaten since at least Roman times. The flavor combines well with carrots and other green vegetables. Snap off the bottom end of the spears and simmer in salted water for up to one-half hour, depending on the spears' thickness, until tender. Cream of asparagus soup makes an especially delectable potion to welcome in the springtime.

Nutrition: Don't throw away the water in which you simmered last night's dinner asparagus; it makes an excellent soup base and facial cleanser. Asparagus water also helps dissolve uric acid deposits and flushes toxins from the kidneys.

Lore: Probably because of the spear-like, phallic shape of the shoots, asparagus is considered an aphrodisiac. Add it to vegetable-based potions to promote passion and fertility.

AVOCADO

(Persea Americana, P. gratissima)

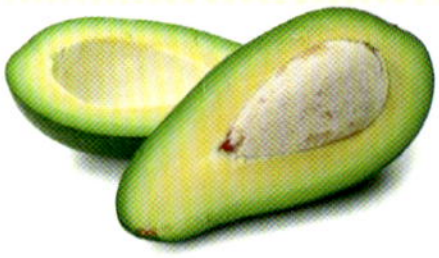

Description: This semi-tropical tree has thrived on the planet so long that prehistoric animals used to feed on them. In the Western Hemisphere, avocados grow from Santa Barbara, California, to Lima, Peru. Six hundred million avocados are harvested every year. You well might ask, "How many of these wonderful fruits go bad in the refrigerator?" After reading this and experimenting with some potion recipes found elsewhere in this book, perhaps you may never consign one of these delightful fruits to the compost bin again. Of the three varieties, the smallest is considered the tastiest, the medium size is the one usually found at the supermarket, and the largest has the mildest flavor and fewest calories.

Culinary Uses: The green or yellowish-green flesh tastes velvety sweet in salads, and also forms the basis of the celebrated Mexican guacamole dip.

Nutrition: Avocados contain a fair amount of potassium. Drinking an avocado potion or eating the fruit helps build facet joints in the vertebrae.

Lore: Because Native Americans from Mexico and Central America used avocados in beauty formulas, this fruit has become a prime ingredient of potions to enhance personal appearance. It also enters into potions to increase fertility and creativity.

BANANA

(Musa genus, especially Musa sapientum, M. paradisiaca)

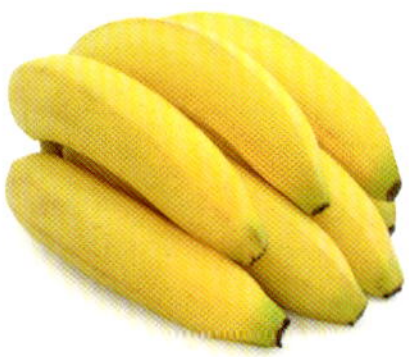

Description: The fruit of this tropical tree is common in markets around the world. It is a native of Asia that was introduced to the Americas by Spanish colonists during the sixteenth century. A Norwegian friend tells us he remembers when bananas first appeared in Norway during the 1950s.

I once thought that only two varieties of bananas existed–the eating banana that we find in most grocery stores in North America and the larger *plátano* that is more fibrous and not as sweet, but fries up well. When I moved to Brazil, I discovered a whole new world of bananas–large and small, white, yellow, and red-fleshed, and with a variety of subtly different flavors. My favorite is the tiny *banana maçã* (apple or silk banana), which, as the name in Portuguese suggests, tastes like an apple.

Culinary Uses: Bananas should not be juiced because they are too soft and fibrous. On the other hand, they make superb blenders for smoothies. Try freezing the banana before you blend it. If the fruit gets overripe, never fear, you can always bake banana bread. This fruit also makes a rich-tasting liqueur.

Nutrition: Bananas contain more pectin than apples and brim with vitamins, including A, B, C, niacin, potassium, riboflavin, thiamine, and fiber. The vitamin K content protects against high blood pressure.

Lore: In Hindu legend, bananas were a forbidden fruit. According to folk superstition, if you make a wish on a banana, peel and eat it, and then find a star-shaped mark at the bottom, your wish will come true. Because the fruit is a phallic-shaped high-energy food, it makes a superb ingredient in potions to promote male energy, sexuality, and fertility.

BEAN

(Phaeolus vulgaris)

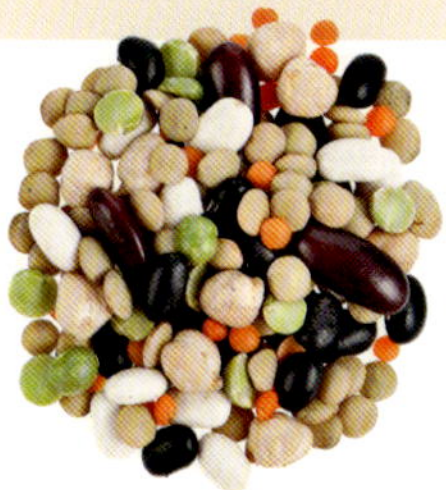

Description: The varieties of beans are almost endless. They include a veritable artist's palette of red, yellow, white, green, black, pink, and cranberry, as well as Anasazi, pinto, shell, bush, snap, lentil, chickpea, popping, soy, lima, runner, fava, dry, and string beans. If you're blending the fresh string, pole, or bush types in potions, select only plump, meaty beans that break with a clean snap when bent. Store in an airtight plastic bag in the refrigerator, or blanch and freeze.

Culinary Uses: When juiced, the bean flavor is strong, so be sure to mix it with a sweeter vegetable like carrot or celery. Any kind of bean can be cooked in a soup, but dry beans such as navy, Anasazi, and pinto types are popular. Wash dry beans thoroughly, transfer to a bowl, and fill the bowl with salt and water. Let the beans soak for a few hours, then wash them, change the water, and soak again overnight before cooking. This process softens the bean and leaches out difficult to digest complex sugars that can cause flatulence.

Soaking is especially important for red kidney beans because they contain concentrated levels of the toxic compound phytohaemagglutinin. To deactivate this toxin you need to soak the beans for at least five hours in water, discard the water, and then boil the beans for ten minutes at 212 degrees Fahrenheit. If you finish cooking the red beans at a lower temperature (176° Fahrenheit or lower, such as in a slow cooker) you run the risk of activating another toxin, haemagglutinin. You know when you've been poisoned if from one to three hours after eating improperly prepared beans, you come down with nausea, vomiting, and diarrhea. Usually the symptoms disappear after a few hours.

Nutrition: Most of the fruits and vegetables listed in this appendix, while full of vitamins and minerals, generally fall down in the protein department. Beans, especially dry varieties, are an exception. Dry beans, like red kidney beans, can contain as much as twenty-four grams of protein per three and one-half ounces. This is why they make great additions to vegetarian and vegan diets. Beans contain vitamins A, B, and C, potassium, zinc, folate, iron, calcium, and magnesium, and offer a lot of fiber. A tea concocted from string bean pods treats diabetes and also promotes weight loss. A word of advice: if you suffer from gout, it is probably a good idea to limit your bean consumption. Beans are high in purine, which converts to uric acid and can irritate your condition.

Lore: The Romans thought that vengeful ghosts threw dried beans at their houses during the night so that bad luck would rain down on the inhabitants. To counteract this possible violence, they cast black beans into the graves of the dead and burned beans during the festival of Lemuri. Nevertheless, they ate the vegetable with reverence as part of their funeral ceremonies. In Greek myth, beans were sacred to the god Apollo and were used in cultures worldwide as a form of divination by sortilege (drawing lots). By analogy they are ingredients for divination potions, especially when a decision about a future action is required.

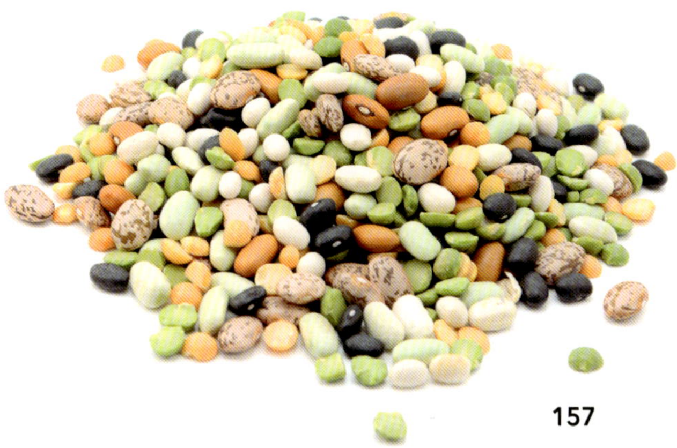

BEET

(Beta vulgaris)

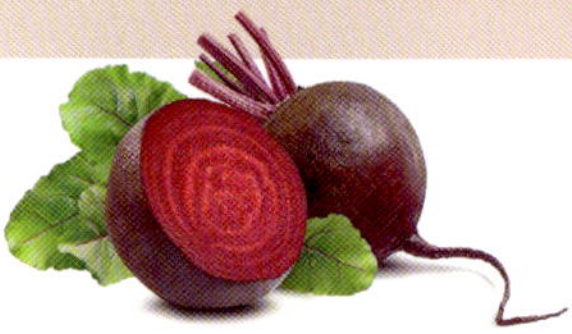

Description: This root crop grows well in cool climates. The two-foot tall plant develops dark green leaves, often veined in red, and a dark red bulb (although some varieties are white or yellow). Choose medium-sized (large beets can be too "woody"), smooth, unblemished roots and store in an airtight plastic bag in your refrigerator or root cellar. One of my favorite varieties is the Detroit Red Beet—perhaps because I grew up in the Detroit area.

Culinary Uses: For juicing, I prefer to use only the bulb, although some cooks add the leaves. The young leaves also make tasty salad greens. In fact, during Roman times, only the leaves were eaten. I advise not to drink beet juice straight because it may irritate your throat and esophagus. Try blending it with milder ingredients such as apples, carrots, or celery. The size, shape, texture, and taste makes the beet a superior pickling vegetable. The popular Russian borscht soup is made with a base of beets. (See recipe in Chapter 12.)

Nutrition: Beets are supercharged with iron. Be aware that when you eat or drink beets, your urine may turn red until the juice has passed from your system.

Lore: The Greeks held this lowly vegetable in such high esteem that they offered it on a silver platter to their god Apollo at the Delphi Temple. Because the taproot is red, the plant is associated with health, passion, and prosperity.

BLACKBERRY

(Rubus fruticosus, R, villosus, R. ursinus)

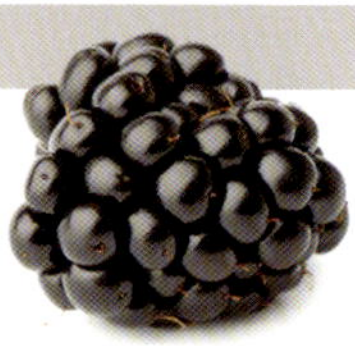

Description: This is not a berry, but an aggregate fruit made up of many tiny fruits. Blackberries grow on a trailing bush that is pricklier than the raspberry bush. Select only firm, deep purple, or jet-black fruit to juice.

Culinary Uses: As with berries, blackberries make tasty jams, jellies, smoothies, wines, pies, and dessert toppings. The dried leaf is a popular and nutritious ingredient of herbal infusions.

Nutrition: Both the fruit and leaf pack a wallop in the nutrition category. Among their nutrients are vitamins C and K, anthocyanin, fiber, folate, magnesium, and manganese. The juice and herbal infusion from the leaves have long been used in herbal medicine to remedy diarrhea. Scientific evidence shows that blackberries are an anti-inflammatory that lowers LDL cholesterol levels and flushes plaque deposits from the arteries. They also combat free radicals in the body, which can lead to various cancers.

Lore: Blackberries are linked to the angel Lucifer who, when he fell to Earth, is alleged to have landed in a blackberry bush. This multi-faceted fruit also belongs to Brigit, the healing goddess of the Irish pantheon. According to legend, if a person suffering any illness on a sunny day crawls backward and forward three times through a bush that has made a natural arch, they will be magically cured. In my opinion, anybody who can do that without getting scratched up doesn't need healing. The leaves and berries are also ingredients of prosperity spells.

BROCCOLI

(Brassica oleracea italica)

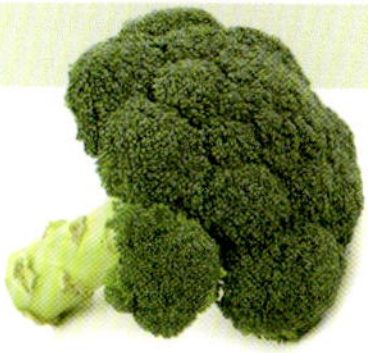

Description: This member of the cabbage family is one of the few vegetables available year-round. It produces bunches of flowering buds on terminal stems as well as on branches; hence its Italian name, which refers to "arms." Look for bunches that smell fresh rather than cabbagy and that have firm (not wiggly) stalks and tightly closed clusters. Avoid yellow-tinged florets (unless you are going for the romanesco variety, which is colored yellowish-green), for this indicates that the plant will taste acrid and dried-out. Wash, dry, and store in an airtight bag in the refrigerator.

Culinary Uses: Until the 1920s, broccoli was eaten mainly by Italian immigrants in the USA, and so was considered an ethnic food. As past President George W. Bush once reminded everyone, broccoli has a strong flavor. So use it sparingly in cooking and juicing, but do use it. Three or four florets are usually enough. I find that if I pour on enough cheese sauce or consume it as broccoli cheese soup, I enjoy the taste very much. (See recipe in Chapter 9.)

Nutrition: You can't fault broccoli on nutrition. A cupful of the fresh florets (without the cheese sauce!) will only set you back thirty calories. As a green food, broccoli is touted as a superb antioxidant. It contains vitamins A and C, small amounts of B6, calcium, iron, and phytochemicals that fight cancer. Recently it has been discovered that broccoli helps with weight loss by balancing hormone levels in the bloodstream.

Lore: In folklore, broccoli is linked to the Roman deity Jupiter. Perhaps because of the way the stalks thrust up from the ground, this plant is added to potions to increase physical and mental stamina, strength, and energy. As such qualities are also sought by people who need to take charge of group situations, broccoli is an ingredient of potions to improve leadership skills. The vegetable is also touted as a male virility enhancer. I suspect this legend came about to encourage guys to quit complaining about the taste and scarf up their vegetables.

CABBAGE

(Brassica oleracea)

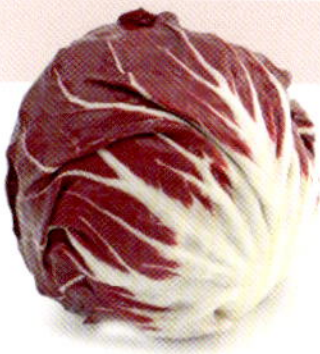

Description: The Latin family name, "crucifer" comes from the word for "cross," and was used to describe the flowers that bloom in the form of a cross. Besides broccoli, which you've already met, other vegetables of the same family include kale, collards, Brussels sprouts, and kohlrabi. They all contain more or less the same nutritional properties.

Cabbage is probably the most ancient cultivated leafy plant. Three major varieties exist: white cabbage, which is the kind you see mainly in the grocery stores with its pale color and smooth, raised veins; savoy, which has wrinkled leaves; and red cabbage, which is like the white variety in shape and size, only with red leaves. (See photo in Chapter 1.) Select heads that are heavy for their size and avoid those with shrunken discolored leaves.

Culinary Uses: Cabbage soup is a staple of Russian and Eastern European cooking. Russian princes used to pay tributes to their kings with plots of land planted with cabbages. Egyptian pharaohs ate plenty of cabbage and drank its juice before embarking on a night of revelry in the belief that they would not get drunk. Perhaps this is the origin of the hangover cure that calls for cabbage juice and vinegar. The strong, sour taste will certainly wake you up! Since the flavor of cabbage juice is so overpowering, I advise you to combine it with a sweeter vegetable like carrot if you are going to juice it. Before placing it in the juicer, cut the head into small wedges.

Nutrition: Cabbage is brimming with vitamins A, C, and K as well as beta-carotene and iron. The juice is a folk remedy for bleeding stomach ulcers. Cabbage contains a chemical which some studies show may lower the risk of lung cancer in smokers. It also is rich in quercetin, a natural antihistamine for allergy sufferers.

Lore: In the *Language of Flowers,* cabbage means "for profit." This prosaic vegetable is considered an aphrodisiac and is added to love potions. In French, the expression *mon petite chue*, "my little cabbage," is a term of endearment. This brassica is also a good luck talisman, at least it was for Babe Ruth. He used to place a leaf under his cap during games and exchange it for a fresh one halfway through. In the legends of some cultures, children were told that babies came from cabbage patches. Perhaps this is the origin of the once-famous Cabbage Patch Doll.

CARROT

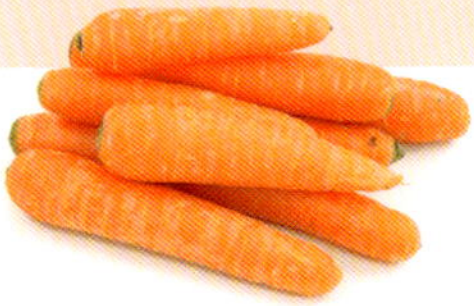

(Daucus carota, D. sativus)

Description: This orange (although other colors exist), long-rooted vegetable is familiar to most. Select roots that are bright-hued and firm with no cracks. Try to purchase organic carrots. If you must buy the non-organic kind, remove the tip and core ends before juicing as this is where pesticides tend to accumulate. Cut the root into two-to-three-inch lengths before juicing.

Culinary Uses: Carrots are now common in gardens and kitchens. They were not considered a food source until relatively recently, although their nutritional and medicinal values have long been recognized. Considering they are a vegetable, carrots contain as much sugar as some fruits. They can sweeten the juices of strong-tasting vegetables like broccoli, cabbage, and cauliflower. However, diabetics should be aware of this fact and avoid them. The carrot flavor combines especially well with apple, celery, cucumber, kale, parsley, pear, spinach, and tangerine.

Nutrition: It's no secret that carrots are good for the eyesight. As an orange food, they are full of beta-carotene, which converts to vitamin A in the body. They also contain a considerable amount of vitamins B-6, niacin, folate, and C, thiamine, manganese, potassium, and of course, fiber. Eating carrots on a regular basis helps regulate the heartbeat and blood pressure and counteracts the negative effects of sodium in the bloodstream. Recent tests with lab rats have shown that carrots destroy pre-cancerous cells and tumors.

Lore: Carrots are said to enhance potions for love, good luck, good sex, and financial gain. They are associated with the planet Mars. At carrot festivals in Scotland, specimens are blessed in the church and returned home to be consumed to bring good health and prosperity to the household. Legend has it that if you're ever unfortunate enough to become possessed by a demon, all you need do is grab a handy carrot and the demon will jump to it. Then, however, you'll have the deep-rooted problem on your hands of how to rid yourself of the possessed carrot!

CAULIFLOWER

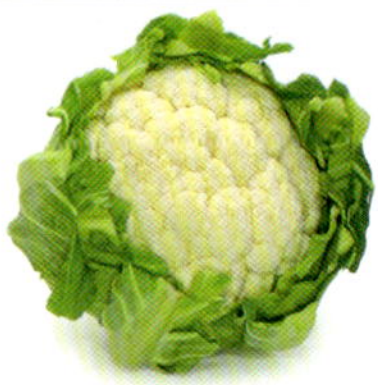

(Brassica oleracea botrytis)

Description: Although this crucifer originated in Asia, it took the Italians to perfect its cultivation. The large, edible, creamy white flower heads are surrounded by green leaves.

Culinary Uses: As with its relatives, broccoli and cabbage, cauliflower juice tastes concentrated, so I recommend only adding a couple of florets to your recipes. Balance the taste by combining with apples or carrots. On the other hand, cauliflower soup tastes buttery and mild, and is a comfort food, especially when served with grated cheese on top. When I lived on the cold, wet, blustery southern coast of Wales, one of my favorite expeditions was to a local lunchroom that served up creamy cauliflower and cheese soup.

Nutrition: Cauliflower has the same nutritional benefits as broccoli and cabbage, listed above. In addition, nibbling on the buds relaxes the blood vessels, which improves the circulation and can help ease headaches.

Lore: The white color of this vegetable relates it to the moon and all of the fascination associated with this heavenly body.

CELERY

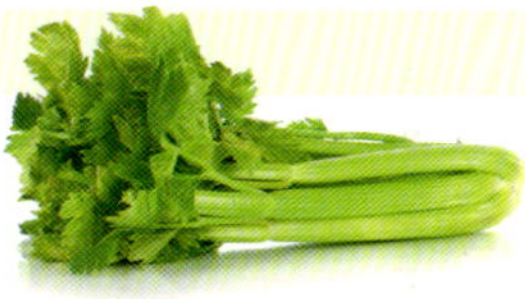

(Apium graveolens)

Description: Although celery's exact origin remains a mystery, this one- to two-foot biennial herb of the carrot family has become naturalized in marshy areas of Europe, especially in the Mediterranean region. Pascal, the most common variety found in grocery stores, has green stalks. The flavor of the ribbed, fleshy, green leafstalk is less pronounced, but they are large, upright, and less stringy than other varieties. Be sure to select stalks that break with a clean snap when you bend them. The leaves should look fresh and bright green in color. Another well-known variety is the self-blanching, yellow celery.

The Latin name for this vegetable means "strong smelling." You may think this odd, as the celery sold at the supermarket has quite a mild aroma and taste. To discover for yourself how densely flavorful true celery is, I recommend growing your own, that is, if you maintain a garden. Celery will also flourish in a large container and does not need full sunlight to grow. In the springtime, garden centers often sell small plants for a couple of dollars. The seeds also germinate easily. I usually start them in a pot and transfer to the garden plot.

Nothing is more delicious than fresh, organic garden-grown celery–supermarket celery doesn't hold a celery stick to it. The flavor is like the difference between winter store-bought tomatoes and summer vine-ripened tomatoes.

Culinary Uses: The seeds and water-filled stalks flavor soups, stews, poultry stuffings, and juices. Celery is easy to juice. Chop it into two-inch lengths before processing.

Nutrition: This veggie contains plenty of vitamins and minerals, including C, B-6, folate, K, riboflavin, calcium, magnesium, manganese, and potassium. Its sodium content is high for a green, leafy vegetable (eighty-eight milligrams per serving), but the sodium is, in part, offset by potassium. Because of the sodium and potassium, drinking a celery-based vegetable drink after a workout helps replace the body's lost electrolytes. Celery is a great diet food because it is low in calories, supplies a lot of fiber, and takes some work to chew and digest. Consuming this vegetable helps alleviate muscle aches and pains, too. Its phytochemical compounds enhance white blood cell production, thereby helping to prevent cancer, and toning the vascular system to treat migraines.

Lore: Celery was one of the holy plants of ancient Greece. Garlands were worn by winners at the Nemean Games in a similar way that bay laurel wreaths festooned Olympic winners. Ancient Romans cooked with celery, but for some unknown reason considered it an unlucky plant to eat, especially on a Tuesday. For centuries, people have chewed celery seeds to aid concentration and grounding. Add the juice of this saturnine vegetable to potions to increase your intuitive abilities and promote beauty, fertility, and love.

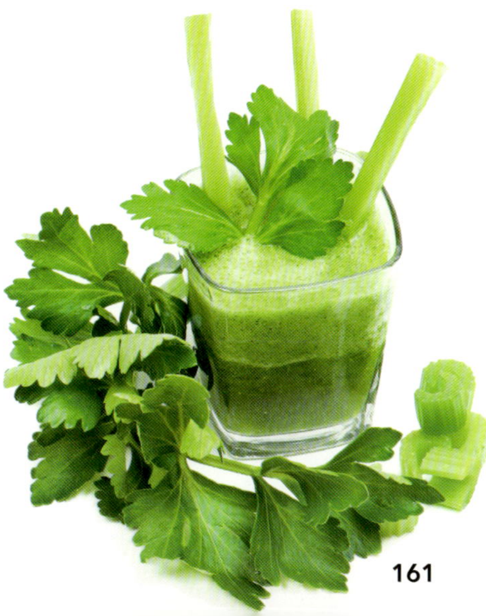

CHERRY

(Prunus avium–Sweet Cherry P. cerasus–Tart Cherry)

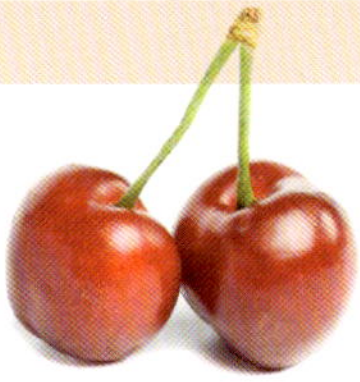

Description: Cherries are the red, dark purplish red, or cream-colored small fruit of a tree grown widely in the temperate zones of the Americas, Europe, and Asia. They ripen earlier than most other tree fruits. The pink blossoms in the springtime are famous for their fragrance and beauty.

Culinary Uses: The juice combines well with carrots, cucumbers, apples, parsley, kale, and tomato. Remove the stone before juicing or blending. Cherry pies and other cherry-flavored desserts are renowned, but if you have the time and inclination, whip up a chilled cherry soup for a summer treat.

Nutrition: Cherries make a superior diet fruit because they satisfy a person's craving for sweets, are fat-free, and help prevent tooth decay. Approximately eighty calories are contained in a cup of sweet cherries and fifty-five in a cup of tart (pie) cherries. Cherry juice treats gout because it dissolves uric acid crystals. The fruit contains fiber and vitamins A, C, and K, calcium, iron, and magnesium. Because tart cherries contain melatonin, they are considered a sleep aid.

Lately, tart cherry juice has been praised as an antioxidant that reduces inflammation in the joints by blocking pain-causing enzymes. The juice also fights heart disease by lowering levels of cholesterol and triglycerides in the blood.

Lore: In the *Language of Flowers,* cherry blossoms symbolize "education." The fragrance is alleged to remove negative influences, encourage light-hearted activities, and create a gay, carefree environment. In the charming old film *The Witches of Eastwick*, cherries are touted as a superior aphrodisiac and fertility enhancer for females. The fruit is also alleged to attract money. For singles yearning to get hitched, here's a divination to do with cherries gleaned from folk superstition. Squeeze a cherry stone between your thumb and forefinger and flick it toward the ceiling. If it hits, you will soon marry.

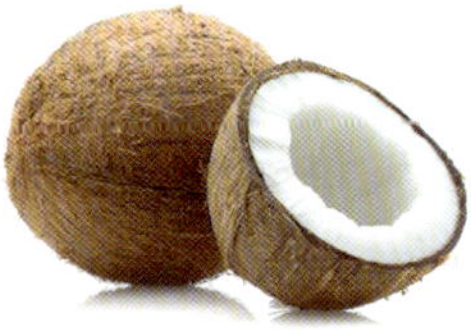

(Cocos nucifera)

Description: This football-size fruit of a palm tree thrives in tropical climates.

Culinary Uses: The oil expressed from the dende palm makes a reasonable substitute for butter. It is an indispensable ingredient in Asian, African, and Afro-Brazilian cooking, imparting a distinctive flavor to those dishes. Coconut milk is not the liquid you find in the middle of the fruit when you crack it open. It is made by shredding the meat and macerating it in hot water, then straining the white cream.

Nutrition: In folk medicine the powdered resin of the fronds of the dende coconut (*Elaeis guinaensis)* treats headaches, angina, diminished vision, leg swelling, and colic. Lately, coconut water has been "discovered" as a low-calorie, natural drink for athletes without the sugar and chemicals found in many sports drinks. See Chapter 6 for information on coconut sugar.

Lore: Coconut signifies "strength in adversity" in the *Language of Flowers,* and is a fruit of Aquarius, the Moon, the Water element, and the Greek goddess Athena. It is associated with potions for beauty, fertility, and gain. Coconut meat, milk, and oil, all symbols of spirituality, are key elements in ritual dishes offered to the deities of the African and Afro-Brazilian pantheons.

CRANBERRY

(Vaccinium macrocarpon)

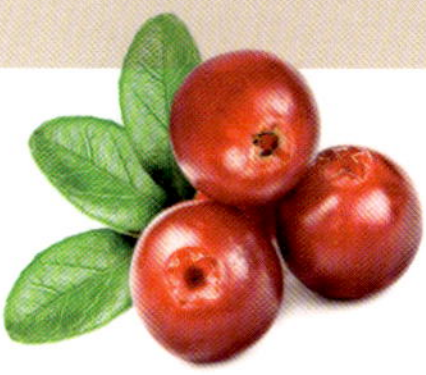

Description: The ruby red berries of this creeping deciduous shrub make a colorful and tangy side dish at the Thanksgiving table, crushed and jellied into a tart sauce to accompany the turkey. The white flowers bloom in snowball clusters on top of leaves that look like maples, although the American colonists thought they looked more like the heads of cranes—hence the plant's name.

Cranberries are usually sold pre-packaged in the supermarket. When you get them home, remove any brown, soft, or mushy berries so they don't contaminate the rest of the fruit. Wash the berries and refrigerate in an airtight plastic bag.

Culinary Uses: The berries reach their peak of ripeness in November and December, which makes them an excellent seasonal choice for holiday dishes. Cranberries are so tart they must have sweetener added to them, or be combined with sweeter juices to taste palatable. The North American Indians used to make a jelly from cranberries prepared with maple sap. I especially like mixing in oranges, walnuts, and apples. Russians serve a cranberry drink called sweet kissel before a meal as an aperitif.

Nutrition: Cranberries are loaded with vitamin C and are good keepers. On long voyages sailors used to store them in barrels to eat to prevent scurvy. Brew a tea from the bark to lessen the pain of childbirth and menstrual cramps and to help alleviate glandular tenderness from mumps. Because cranberries contain a tannin that inhibits bacterial growth in the urinary tract, you can nip a bladder infection in the bud by drinking a large glass of cranberry juice every two hours. The antioxidants in cranberries help prevent dental plaque and guard against cancer.

A word of caution: if you take a blood thinner or suffer from kidney stones, doctors advise you to eliminate cranberries from your diet.

Lore: Colonists were introduced to this fruit by Native Americans, who considered the berries a symbol of peace and protection. Because of its bright red color, this fruit is linked to Mars (the red planet) and Sagittarius (a fire sign). Juice them in potions for protection, especially for safety in travel.

CUCUMBER

(Cucumis sativus)

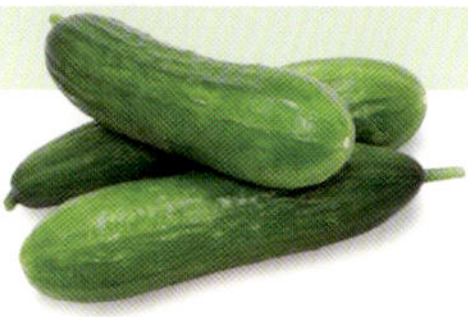

Description: The Latin name means "green grower." Cucumber is a warm-weather plant. Its long, slightly lumpy, green-skinned, water-filled fruit is probably familiar to most. Some varieties are yellow and some taste like lemons. Cukes are native to India, where they have been cultivated for 3,000 years. If you can't grow your own, be sure to buy slender, bright green-colored fruit that is firm with no sign of wrinkling. Shriveled cukes taste bitter.

Culinary Uses: Cold, cucumber soup makes a refreshing treat during hot summer weather. The juice combines well with carrots, celery, and parsley. To juice, peel away the skin, and cut into small chunks.

Nutrition: Cucumbers are rich in vitamins A, C, and K, folate, and a variety of minerals, chief among them, silica. The cooling juice has been used to cure eye infections, sunburn, and dermatitis. Slices of cold cucumber on the eyelids reduces redness and puffiness.

Lore: Because they contain so much water, the *Doctrine of Signatures* associates cucumbers with the moon, the "watery" planet. In Ancient Rome, women who wished to conceive would walk around with a cucumber attached to their waists. The seeds are used in potions as an aphrodisiac and to gain fertility and love as well as for intuitive self-development and divination. In the *Language of Flowers,* this plant inexplicably means "criticism." The term "cool as a cucumber" has led the superstitious to believe that cucumbers possess the power to kill, especially for revenge, because they are so cold. Naturally, this is all nonsense.

CURRANT

(Ribes nigrum)

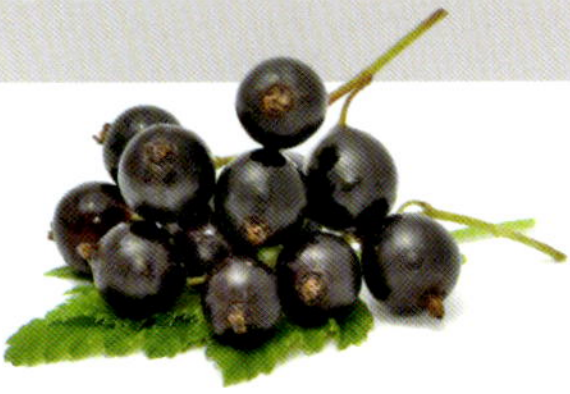

Description: Although a red variety exists, the black currant is more common. Currants are harvested from a perennial woodland shrub.

Culinary Uses: The tart berries mark a cornerstone of British baking, while Americans tend to use raisins instead. The British use currants to flavor everything from scones to cakes and puddings. Maybe that's because they realize how healthy currants are for you. This fruit also is a principale ingredient of Cassis liqueur.

Nutrition: Most fruits and vegetables provide nutrition, but the tiny currants are exceptionally valuable. They weigh in at only seventy-two calories per cup and are replete with calcium, vitamin C, magnesium, zinc, phosphorous, and a chemical called anthocyanoside, which clears away plaque from the arteries, promotes blood vessel strength, and helps stave off age-related vision problems. The sweetened juice known colloquially as "Rob," is gargled as a home remedy for sore throat. It is also drunk to bring down a fever and detoxify the system through its diuretic action. Currants are deemed to strengthen one's resistance to colds and flu and to help mitigate night blindness. Recent studies have shown that this fruit may keep Alzheimer's disease at bay.

Lore: In the *Language of Flowers* this botanical "pleases everyone." It can be used in prosperity potions and formulas to solidify friendships.

FIG

(Ficus carica)

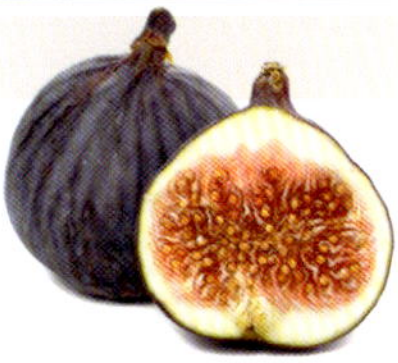

Description: Figs belong to the mulberry family. The fruit grows on vines, shrubs, and trees, and many varieties exist worldwide. Two basic kinds available in the US are the golden brown-colored fig and the purplish black variety. In recent years, several cold hardy varieties have been developed. I admit to being skeptical about this, so I kept my fig in a large container and moved it indoors for the winter. Slowly it lost its leaves, and then put out shoots again in the early spring. For the last two years I've kept it planted outdoors with some protection. The first year it almost died, but is doing nicely now.

When buying figs, choose firm, fragrant fruit and peel them before processing.

Culinary Uses: I admit it: figs are one of my favorite fruits (hence, the reason I keep a bush). Unfortunately, they don't juice well on their own because the flesh is so dense. Try combining them with apple juice, ice cream, or milk for a delicious fig smoothie. Or use candied figs and fig compote in your potion recipes.

Nutrition: Even though they pack a hefty forty calories for their small size, figs decrease the appetite. So unless you overdose, they may help you lose weight. The Japanese have isolated a chemical in figs called benzaldehyde, which is so effective against cancer that it is being added to some cancer-fighting medicines. In Brazil, a tea made from the leaves of some varieties is taken to alleviate the symptoms of intestinal and stomach disorders and aid digestion.

Lore: Figs have acquired something of a split personality in the world of myth and lore. Some traditions claim this fruit is the true elixir of life. Eating figs, they say, will give the face a youthful glow and increase longevity. In other legends, the fruit is cursed. In the Bible (Matthew 21:19), Jesus said, "'Let there be no more fruit from you forever,' And the fig tree immediately dried up." Actually, Jesus was referring in symbolic terms to the religious systems of the time. Nonetheless, this dual attitude is shown by the fact that figs have been associated with a wide variety of ancient deities, including Dionysus, Pan, Artemis, Jupiter, Thoth, Isis, and in the Brazilian pantheon with Xangô, the Thunder God, Nanã, the grandmother goddess, and Exu, the trickster. Plato remarked that figs are the philosopher's best friend, so he may have thought they conferred wisdom.

GRAPE

(Vitis vinifera)

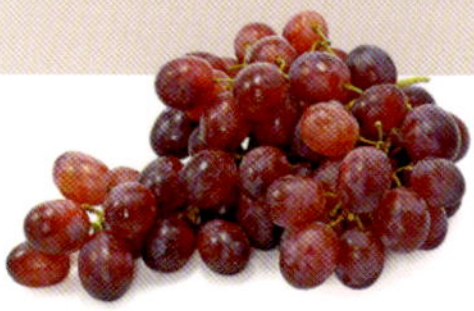

Description: Grapes grow in clusters on woody vines. Colors vary from golden to green, red, and purple. There is evidence that grapes have been cultivated for 8,000 years, which makes them the oldest and probably most widely cultivated fruit worldwide. Types include those grown for eating (table grapes), winemaking, and raisins. Buy the table varieties for juicing, as they are plumpest. More than any other fruit, I recommend you buy organic grapes because non-organic crops are heavily sprayed with pesticides.

Culinary Uses: Wash grapes thoroughly and remove the stems, but not the skins before juicing.

Nutrition: While all grapes are blessed with vitamins A, B, C, K, calcium, iron, manganese, and zinc, the red variety is considered the most nutritious. Resveratrol, plentiful in both grape juice and red wine, has received a lot of press in recent years for its capacity to reduce coronary heart disease, inhibit growth of cancerous tumors, and help increase the lifespan.

Lore: In Christianity grapes are a symbol of the blessed Eucharist and the juice is drunk during communion as the blood of Christ. Voodun practitioners swear that the scent of grapes pulls in money and popularity and shrugs off curses. Like most fruit, they are an ingredient of fertility potions and potions to prompt visions of the future.

In the *Language of Flowers* grapes stand for "charity." In ancient Greece, grapes were sacred to Dionysus, and to Bacchus in Rome. In fact, there were cults to these gods, who symbolized inspiration. By analogy, grape juice potions are drunk today to gain inspiration and strengthen the mind. Because grapes grow in clusters, they go into potions to bring together in unity and peace people who hold differences of opinion.

GRAPEFRUIT

(Citrus paradise)

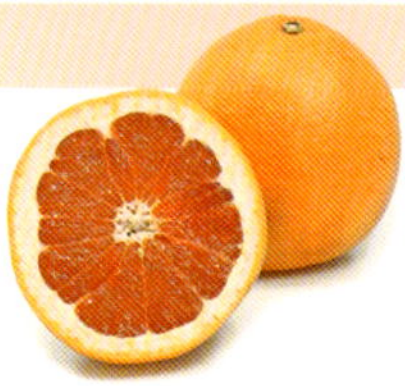

Description: Grapefruit is a citrus fruit that looks like an orange, only larger. It grows in clusters like grapes (hence, its name) on semi-tropical and tropical trees. The flesh is yellow or orange in color, and tangy to sour tasting. Along with other citrus trees, Columbus brought grapefruit to the New World, where they have become naturalized. In the US, trees are cultivated mainly in Florida and Texas. When buying grapefruit, select a smooth-skinned fruit from a green (not brown) stem that is round, plump, fragrant, and heavy for its size. Refrigerate and wash thoroughly before juicing.

Culinary Uses: Since grapefruit can taste sour, the juice combines best with sweeter fruits such as apple and orange. When juicing, remove the skin, but leave the pith. One interesting way to eat grapefruit is to make a syrup from the juice, combined with red wine and sweetener.

Nutrition: Grapefruit helps prevent heart disease by lowering LDL cholesterol levels. It also curbs hunger. Since each fruit weighs in at a mere thirty-to-thirty-five calories, it's a heaven-sent treat for dieters. The salicylic acid content helps mitigate arthritis pain and the lycopene in grapefruit guards against cancerous tumors and free radicals. The seed extract remedies sore throat and bacterial infections.

Lore: This fruit is so nutritious it has become a principal ingredient of better health and physical protection potions as well as potions for spiritual purification.

JICAMA

(Pachyrhizus erosus)

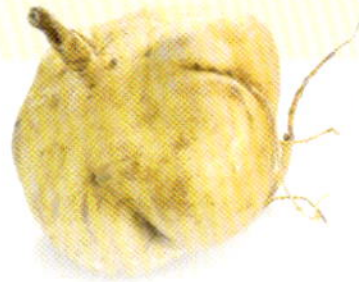

Description: The large, tuberous root of this leguminous vegetable is the part eaten. Peel away the brown skin to reveal a yellowish-white flesh that tastes slightly nutty sweet, like a cross between a chestnut and an apple. Buy roots that are firm, but not too big.

Culinary Uses: This major crop of Mexico appears as an ingredient in many traditional dishes. Jicama combines well with other vegetables. Remove the skin and cut it into cubes before juicing.

Nutrition: The root is a good source of vitamins C and B complex and various minerals, including calcium and phosphorus. It is a source of Inulin, a zero-calorie dietary fiber that does not metabolize, thereby making jicama a dieter's choice for sweet snacking.

Lore: Jicama is a component of potions designed to increase virility and fertility in males–and it tastes a heck of a lot better than Viagra!

LEMON

(Citrus limon)

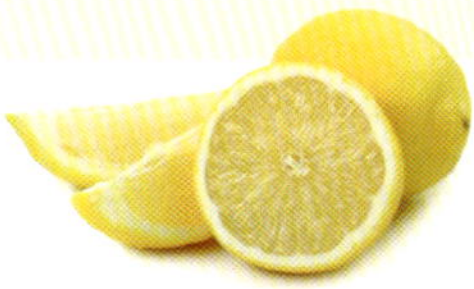

Description: The pale, yellow, acidic fruit of this tropical citrus tree has been cultivated in India for 2,500 years. I have found patio lemons easy to grow in pots. I bring them indoors during the winter and keep them in a north-facing window. The lemons are somewhat smaller and milder than store-bought, but nothing beats harvesting your own organic lemons in the middle of a Colorado winter.

Culinary Uses: Lemons add zest to many dishes and drinks, especially the more flat-tasting green and herbal teas. Since they are so sour, this is one case where I recommend you add sweetener to make lemonade.

Here's a trick I picked up living in Brazil for buying fresh, juicy lemons. When I go to the outdoor market, I avoid lemons with coarse skin and a deep yellow color, as they are probably old lemons that yield less juice. I pick up a likely candidate and roll it lightly between my thumb and forefinger to estimate the juiciness. You can do the same thing with limes, but not with oranges. Some potion recipes require lemon zest, which is merely grated lemon peel.

Nutrition: Lemons purify the blood because they are diuretic. This is why drinking a glassful of water with the juice from a slice or two of lemon in the morning is good for cleaning out your system. Take care not to drink lemon juice in a concentrated dose, as it can eat away tooth enamel. My advice is to drink the lemon water before brushing your teeth to brush away remaining acid.

Lore: The lemon tree is associated with the sun and the element Fire, probably because it looks like a big yellow orb. Consume lemon juice in potions to contact otherworldly planes of existence, promote beauty and longevity, and stimulate joy. A few drops in any potion increases its power. Lemons refresh and stimulate the mind, but also relax nervous, overly talkative people. If you want to get your point across at the dinner table without a lot of interruption, serve lemonade. Naturally, this botanical signifies "zest" in the *Language of Flowers*.

LETTUCE

(Lactuca sativa)

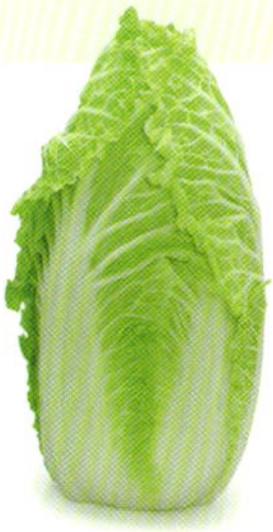

Description: Many varieties of this leafy vegetable exist, but the main difference is between those that form heads and those that remain leafy. Typical kinds of grocery store lettuce include butter, head, Boston, bibb, and romaine.

Since lettuce grows close to the ground, I recommend buying organically grown produce. Select heads with crisp leaves that smell like a fresh morning garden; avoid wilted leaves and oversized heads. When you get your lettuce home, rinse it thoroughly in cold water or soak it for a few minutes in a pot of water to remove clinging dirt. Take the lettuce from the pot and shake it to remove the water. Wrap loosely in paper or a cloth towel and refrigerate.

Culinary Uses: Most lettuce tastes sweet and will tone down strong-flavored juices like cabbage, cauliflower, and broccoli. Loose-leaf varieties are not as good for juicing because the leaves are so thin. To juice, fold a few leaves into a ball and place them in the juicer. Lettuce combines well with carrots and celery.

Nutrition: This leafy vegetable is rich in vitamins A, B, C, E, calcium, iron, and magnesium.

Lore: The Egyptians believed that lettuce was an aphrodisiac, yet in the *Language of Flowers* it means "cold-hearted." Makes you wonder what occurred between Egyptian and Victorian times to create such an about-face. This vegetable is also consumed in potions to create a feeling of peace and harmony and to draw prosperity. After all, if you are feeling at one with the universe, you are truly prosperous.

LIME

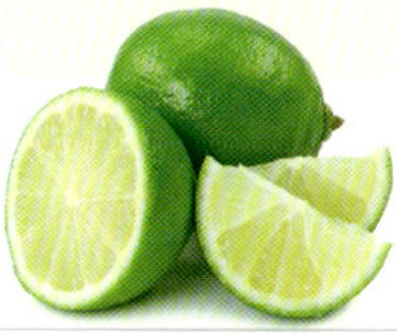

(Citrus aurantifolia)

Description: Limes are similar to lemons, only smaller, with a thinner, tighter skin. They are dark green in color and are more aromatic and less acidic than lemons. Limes grow on spiny shrubs in tropical areas around the world such as India, Mexico, Brazil, and the West Indies.

Culinary Uses: In tropical regions, limes often replace lemons in cooking. The flavor is so distinctive that lemons never quite manage to replace the lime's unique tartness. Limes are an essential ingredient of the popular Mexican alcoholic drink, the margarita. In Brazil beach vendors sell a wonderful non-alcoholic concoction made from mate tea, ginger, and lime called *mate-limão*. Brazil's most famous alcoholic drink, the *caipirinha,* is a small drink made with freshly squeezed lime, local sugarcane liquor, ice, and a blizzard of fast-dissolving sugar.

Nutrition: As with all citrus fruits, limes contain vast quantities of vitamin C. British sailors used to suck on them when they went on long voyages to stave off scurvy. Eventually, those sailors became known as "limeys."

Lore: Lime makes a perfect choice for cleansing and purification potions.

MANGO

(Mangifera indica)

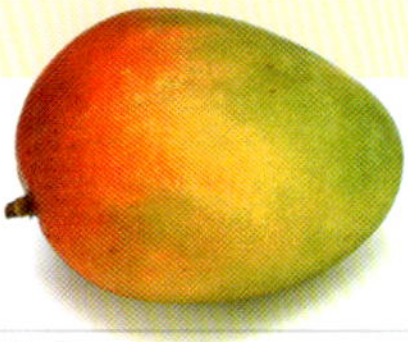

Description: This spreading tree native to India flourishes throughout tropical regions. The fruit has a greenish, yellowish, or reddish skin. The flesh on the inside is as orange as a carrot, thick and pulpy and overflowing with juice.

Culinary Uses: Mangos are one of my favorite fruits. As a child living in Mexico City, I used to carry a mango in my lunch box every day. I remember riding on the school bus eating my mango, not minding at all that sticky juice ran down my chin and onto my clothes because the fruit was so sweet. Mango sorbet is one of the true pleasures of the gastronomical world as is the Indian delight, mango *lassi*. Remove the skin and the enormous seed before juicing.

Nutrition: The orange pulp is a giveaway that this fruit is high in beta-carotene. It also contains vitamin C, iron, plenty of fiber, and natural fruit sugar for energy. Syrup concocted from the pulp soothes bronchitis and the juice extracted from the branches counteracts diarrhea. Mangos are said to combat body odor, so you can be healthy and odor-free if you eat lots of mangos.

Lore: A legend about the Mango Princess claims that if you meet her in the forest, you will learn the true nature of the Self. In Asia, this fruit is sacred to Buddha because he meditated in a mango grove. Sip mango juice on a hot afternoon, lean back in your shaded hammock, and meditate on the power and purpose of your life. Mangos also go into prosperity and happiness potions.

MELON

(Cucurbitaceae family)

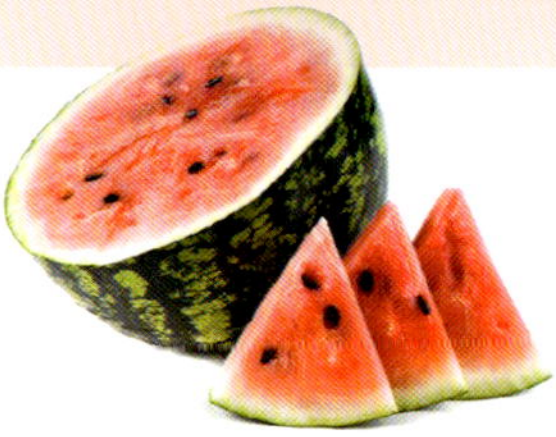

Description: Melons include several varieties of large, gourd-like, juicy fruit that grow on trailing vines. The beta-carotene content of melons gives them their colors, which range from red to orange, yellow, and green. When selecting melons, look for those that smell fresh at the stem end, are bruise-free, and feel heavy for their size. Store at room temperature. If you must refrigerate, wrap them in cellophane so they don't absorb refrigerator odors.

Culinary Uses: With their distinctive perfume melons transform a plain fruit salad into ambrosia. Their flavor combines well with any kind of berry in a juice. As their name implies, watermelons are comprised of ninety-one percent water, and so make an excellent choice for juicing.

Nutrition: The healthy content of melons includes beta-carotene, which bolsters the immune system and the blood coagulater vitamin K. Melons are low in calories, the highest being the cantaloupe, which weighs in at fifty-seven per cup. The lowest is honeydew with a mere thirty-three calories per cup.

Lore: Like gourds, the heavy, water-filled melons are associated with the moon, which traditionally stands for intuition, creativity, and fertility. One unusual superstition about melons has been handed down by the Romani. They say that if you keep a melon or even a pumpkin in the house too long, it will begin to move and make noises. I've been staring at my Thanksgiving cornucopia decoration, which includes melons, and has graced the dining table for more than a month. So far, I've only detected movement when a family member swipes a melon to eat.

MUSHROOM

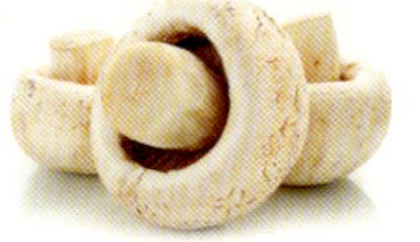

(Common mushroom: Agaricus bisporus)

Description: The term "mushroom" refers to the fruit of different species of fungi, gilled or not gilled, with or without stems, cultivated or wild. The *Agarocus bisporus* or white button variety is the most familiar sight at the grocery. Over the last few years, more cultivated varieties are showing up such as the maitake (hen-of-the-woods), shitake, Portobello, and morel. In popular jargon, "toadstools" refer to poisonous mushrooms. For example, the *Amarita phalloides* death cap has been popularized in murder mysteries. Psychedelic-hallucinogenic mushrooms, known as magic mushrooms and shrooms, are a big hit with the druggie crowd.

I suggest you either grow your own or buy them in the grocery store because it is dangerous to forage in the wild for mushrooms. Every year a few people die as a result of eating poison mushrooms that they collect on their own. In spite of modern medicine's best efforts, there is no cure for mushroom poisoning.

Culinary Uses: Mushrooms don't juice well, but you can cook them in butter or olive oil and add them to soups, sauces, and stuffing. Their delicate flavor is enhanced by adding garlic.

Nutrition: For a long time it was assumed that mushrooms offered no nutrients. Lately they have been discovered to provide phosphorous, niacin, zinc, and small amounts of riboflavin, protein, and pantothenic acid. Studies have been performed in Japan on the medicinal value of mushroom extract with the possibility of using it as an antiviral, antibacterial, immune system and heart strengthener, and tumor blaster. Be advised that mushrooms readily absorb heavy metals. Radioactive mushrooms have been discovered near Chernobyl since the failure of that nuclear reactor.

Lore: Our ancestors believed that mushrooms, which are associated with the Moon, made superior love and fertility potions. In Ancient Egypt, they were called the "plant of immortality." In the *Language of Flowers* this vegetable stands for "suspicion," possibly because it is so difficult to distinguish the poisonous ones from the non-poisonous varieties. In the mythology of the Celtic cultures rings of mushrooms were thought to be fairy circles. If a person perchance ventured inside one of these rings, the fairies would take them to visit strange and exotic locales. Add mushrooms to potions for personal growth and communication with fairies or the Little People.

ORANGE

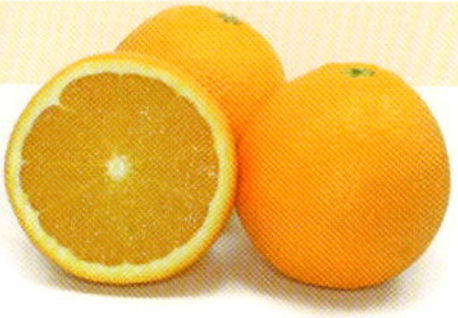

(Citrus aurantium, C. sinensis)

Description: This large, round, orange-colored fruit from a tropical citrus tree is so popular it probably needs no description. Sweet oranges were unknown in Europe until 1498 when Portuguese explorer Vasco da Gama brought them back from his trip around Cape of Good Hope.

Navel oranges are so named for the navel-like button on the end opposite the stem. They are juicy, seedless, and easy to peel. Temple and Seville oranges are tart, but good in desserts. Moro and blood oranges are juicy, with the blood orange being slightly sweeter and strawberry-raspberry flavored. Valencia oranges are especially good to juice because they contain few seeds.

Culinary Uses: Oranges flavor creams, cakes, jams, sauces, custards, and a variety of sweet dishes, as well as popular liqueurs like Grand Marnier and Cointreau. Before juicing, remove the peel and cut into wedges.

Nutrition: Oranges are renowned for their high vitamin C and calcium content. The thiamine (a B vitamin) in the fruit helps deliver oxygen to the body. Oranges also contain potassium, a mineral that helps your body achieve electrolyte balance. Pregnant women might want to drink the juice, which is rich in folic acid, an important element for fetal brain development. The antioxidants in orange juice are the kind that help cure rheumatism, pneumonia, and arthritis. They also help alcoholics break their addiction. Orange blossom tea purifies the digestive system. Orange flavoring goes down well with most children, so the juice is a good way to persuade them to drink up their daily health potions.

Lore: In Greek legend one of Zeus's marriage gifts to Hera was an orange. Brides still wear orange blossoms on their wedding day to ensure a long, happy, fertile marriage. Give an orange to your lover to draw you closer together. In the *Language of Flowers* orange blossoms stand for "chastity" and "generosity." Add orange peel to your arsenal of potion ingredients to cultivate a love partner. Include the juice of any kind of orange in potions to attract a mate and keep your lover faithful. Because oranges encourage people to open up, an orange-based punch makes a perfect icebreaker for social occasions. (See recipe in Chapter 17.)

PAPAYA

(Carica papaya)

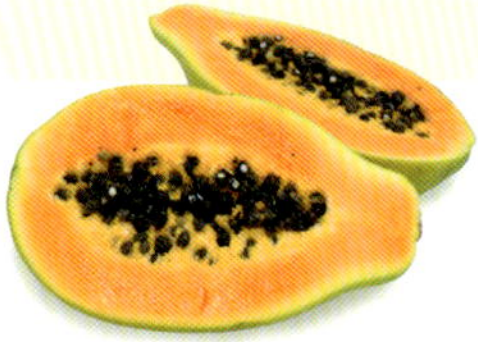

Description: This fruit is known as a Papaw in some countries, but in the US, another fruit goes by that name. The slightly elongated, green papaya hangs like a melon under a crown of leaves atop a single scarred stem. The fruit looks a little like a large pear with patches of light orange or yellow. The flesh is a salmon-apricot color. Inside is a hollow center filled with black seeds suspended in grayish gelatin. Look for a fruit that appears heavy for its size and that gives slightly when you apply pressure to the skin. Spots on the skin do not affect the flavor.

Culinary Uses: Not only does the flesh look like an apricot, it tastes somewhat apricot-like, only muskier with peachy overtones. A milky substance that exudes from the fruit is used to manufacture chewing gum. The edible seeds have a pungent taste similar to mustard. To juice, cut the fruit in half, peel away the skin, and scoop out the seeds. Cooks in tropical lands wrap meat in papaya leaves to tenderize it.

Nutrition: Papaya contains most of the nutrients we have come to associate with fruit such as vitamins A, C, and E, beta-carotene, calcium, potassium, manganese, phosphorous, and iron. Papain enzyme, named for the plant, helps break down fats and stimulates the kidneys. Papain can digest one thousand times its weight in proteins and carbohydrates. It also contains citric and malic acids that help flush away fat.

Lore: There is a superstition among the older generation of Thai people that warns against planting a papaya tree in the garden or it will rain bad luck on the home. This story probably originated because papayas are easily uprooted and people didn't want a tree falling on the house. This superstition aside, papaya is an ingredient of potions for love, prosperity, and good health. As an orange food, it is ideal in smoothies to sharpen the intellect.

PASSION FRUIT

(Passiflora incarnata)

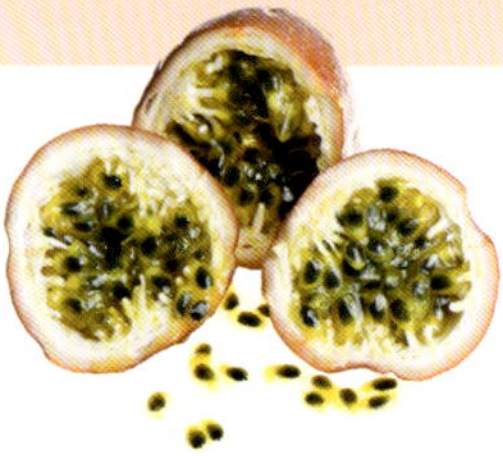

Description: Christians see in the features of the purple flowers of this climbing vine the symbols of the Crucifixion, hence its name. The corona in the center resembles a crown of thorns. The tendrils symbolize the cords that bound Jesus to the Cross. The three stigmas seem like the nails with which He was hung on the Cross. The leaves, to some, look like the thirty pieces of silver for which He was betrayed. The bud represents the Eucharist; the half-open flowers, the Star of the East; the five stamens, the Five Wounds; and finally, the ten petals, the Ten Apostles minus Peter and Judas.

Culinary Uses: Some species bear an egg-shaped fruit. The skin is hard, thick, and wrinkled, but oh what sweet flavor awaits within the golden-colored flesh! The seeds are edible as well. Choose a fruit that is shriveled and fragrant. If the skin is still smooth, ripen it at room temperature. Wash and store in an airtight plastic bag in the refrigerator. Before juicing, cut the fruit in half. There is no need to remove the seeds.

Nutrition: As an antispasmodic, nervine, and sedative, passion fruit restores frazzled nerves and helps cure insomnia. Because it has a narcotic action, it has been used effectively to mitigate the pain of various neurological diseases. Be aware that this botanical can cause irregular heartbeat, dizziness, and confusion, so take care when giving it to somebody in an infusion.

Lore: The flower and fruit are alleged to bring good luck in love and are supposed to make an indifferent lover burn with passion. This is probably due to confusion between the words "passion" with a small "p" and "Passion" with a capital "P." This botanical represents "belief," "susceptibility," and "superstition" in the *Language of Flowers*. In mythology it is associated with the sun and Neptune. Add passion fruit to potions to bless the home and overcome fear of public speaking.

PEA

(Pisum sativum)

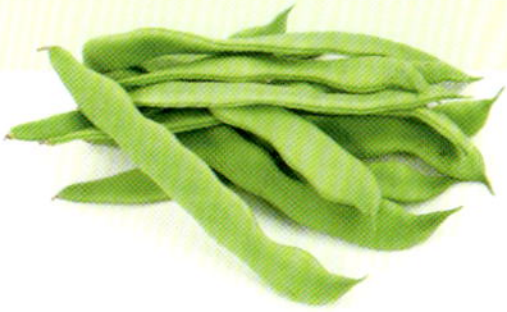

Description: Little round green peas grow in shells on trailing vines. Crops do especially well in cool climates. Many varieties exist, including snow, green, and sugar snap peas.

Culinary Uses: Add whole peas to soups and salads, and enjoy them as a colorful vegetable accompaniment to a meal. Pea soup with ham, bread, and cheese on the side makes a hearty winter meal. Peas can also be put through the blender. The water in which they have been boiled can be used as a base for other soups. Be aware that pea soup is slightly laxative.

Nutrition: This vegetable rich in vitamins A, B-6, C, niacin, and K, carotene, phosphorous, thiamin, copper, and manganese. Unlike some vegetables, peas also contain a good deal of protein. They help dissolve blood clots and increase the circulation. The water in which they have been boiled can be made into a poultice to clear rashes from measles, chickenpox, and eczema.

Lore: The Greeks and Romans considered the innocuous pea an instigator of unruly conduct because of the way it grows with wild abandon on the vine. Formerly, in Britain on Passion Sunday, peas were cooked steeped in butter and given away as an act of charity. They are a prosperity potion ingredient. (See recipe in Chapter 17.)

PEACH AND NECTARINE

(Prunus persica; Prunus persica, var. nectarine)

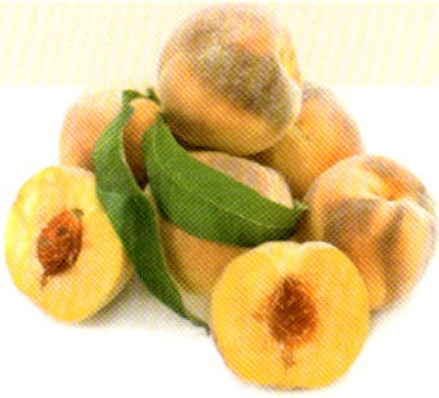

Description: Peach trees form an abundant supply of snowy spring flowers followed by a luscious crop of yellow or rosy-colored fruit in July through September. Two main types include cling peaches, where the stone clings to the flesh, and freestone peaches, where it is easily removed. The color does not necessarily indicate ripeness as some varieties just happen to turn to a rosy blush when ripe. Nectarines are a smooth-skinned variety. A ripe peach yields gently to the touch. This fruit will keep in the refrigerator for several days.

Culinary Uses: Like apples, peaches make fantastic pies, dessert fillings, and jam. They can also be pureed after removing the stone.

Nutrition: Peaches contain relatively few calories for a fruit–only sixty per cup–and have a lot of fiber, so they are considered a dieter's friend. The phytonutrients inhibit cancerous tumor growth. Besides the usual vitamins and minerals associated with most fruit, peaches contain the carotenoids, lutein and zeaxanthin, which help protect the macula of the eye from degenerating. Blend peaches with milk and oatmeal for a refreshing beauty smoothie potion. Peach juice helps eradicate shingles and psoriasis. The kernels are blended commercially in medicinal syrups to reduce fevers and congestion from the flu and help expel intestinal parasites.

Lore: In the *Language of Flowers* the peach blossom signifies "you're terrific" and "I am your captive." (Maybe that's the subconscious reason I named my prettiest kitty Peaches.) The fruit is venerated in China as one of the "fairy fruits" or "fruits of immortality." So it makes sense to add peaches to longevity and anti-depression potions. According to Chinese legend, the most auspicious time for marriage is in February, when peach trees bloom in that country. The peach was so revered there in ancient times that Taoist priests made seals and talismans from the wood. To dream of peaches betides good health, pleasure, and contentment.

PEAR

(Pyrus communis)

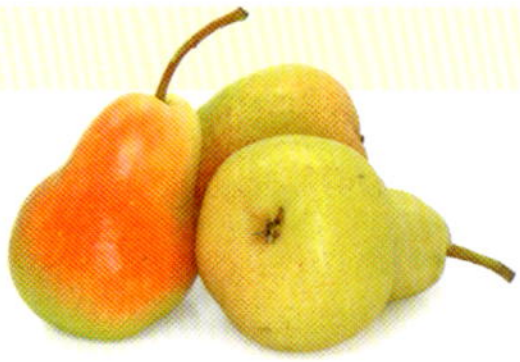

Description: The pear tree is native to Western Asia and Southern Europe and has been cultivated for millennia. This member of the rose family comes in an incredible 3,000 varieties and produces fragrant spring blossoms. At the grocery store you generally find Bartlett (bell-shaped), Bosc (rough on the outside with a long neck and rust-red color), concorde, cornice, red and green Anjou, and Asian varieties like Fuji. Pears ripen from the inside out and ripen best after harvesting. This is why the fruit you buy in the grocery store is so hard and needs to mature in a brown paper bag at room temperature.

Culinary Uses: Pear juice serves multiple functions in cooking because it is so sweet. It tends to be rather thick, so I recommend you cut it with a thinner juice such as apple.

Nutrition: The fruit brims with vitamins A, B complex, C, and E., folic acid, copper, phosphorous, iron (some varieties), and pectin, a soluble fiber that helps flush away cholesterol.

Lore: In the *Language of Flowers* pear means "affection," "give me some hope," and "comfort." According to folk superstition, drinking the juice is said to remove succubae and obsessed spirits from a person's aura. I prefer to think of pear juice as sucking out all the bad cholesterol from my body. The pear is also considered an oracular fruit because in the Old Testament the pear tree gave David the signal to attack the Philistines. Scots will tell you that the true isle of Avalon is actually an island in Argyle shire where blessed pear trees grow wild. The fruit is sacred to the goddesses Venus and Athena. Drink pear juice as a potion for good fortune, longevity, happiness–and simply because it's so sweet!

PEPPER

(Capiscum species)

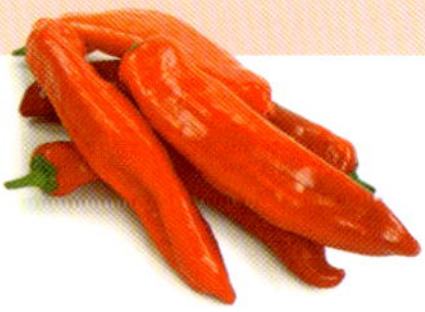

Description: Out of the scores of peppers that exist, the type I focus on in this appendix is the sweet American bell pepper because it is the one most often used in juicing. Hot cayenne pepper is treated in Chapter 6. Bell peppers can be green, red, or yellow, or even purplish-black. Select one with a glossy sheen not produced artificially by wax. Make sure it is firm and without brown spots. Wash and refrigerate until ready to use and remove the seeds before juicing. An interesting bit of trivia is that the pepper king Elihu Yale founded Yale University with the money he made from growing peppers.

Culinary Uses: Sweet peppers are a versatile, crisp vegetable that perk up salads. They are also tasty when stuffed and roasted, or eaten in soups, stews, or pasta sauces. The fruits can be harvested at any time, but the sweetest flavor develops fully at maturity. Peppers blend well with stronger flavored vegetables.

Nutrition: Peppers help stop bleeding and dissolve blood clots, lower blood sugar and cholesterol levels, keep the heart healthy, and help prevent cataracts.

Lore: Red peppers are alleged to drive off the devil, probably because of their fiery color. In ancient Rome, they were thought to be an antidote for hemlock poisoning. The Greeks also considered the pepper a symbol of high rank. Blend sweet peppers in potions for happiness. In the *Language of Flowers* pepper stands for "send me an answer."

PERSIMMON

(Diospyros virginiana)

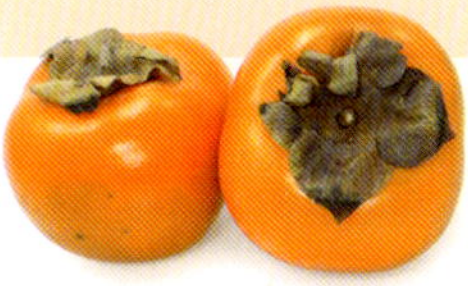

Description: The genus name means "Fruit of the Gods." Persimmons probably originated in China, where they have been cultivated for centuries. The shape of the fruit can be round, square, flattened, or acorn-like. The color varies from light yellow to orange and dark, reddish-orange. Select a fruit with a slightly wrinkled skin. Contrary to other fruit, the best tasting persimmons are those that look like they are on the verge of spoiling. Frost enhances the flavor.

Culinary Uses: If unripe, the taste is sour, but sweetens on ripening. All parts are edible except for the seed and calyx. Remove them before juicing and cut the fruit into quarters.

Nutrition: Persimmon is an astringent that helps cure vaginal yeast infections and intestinal worms. Its antioxidant components help impair cancerous tumors.

Lore: Use in potions for success, passion, fertility, and energy. According to weather folklore, you can predict winter's severity by cutting a persimmon seed in half and observing the shape inside. If it looks like a knife, it will be cold and windy; if it resembles a shovel, resign yourself to shoveling a lot of wet snow. Look out, Punxsutawney Phil!

PINEAPPLE

(Ananas comosus)

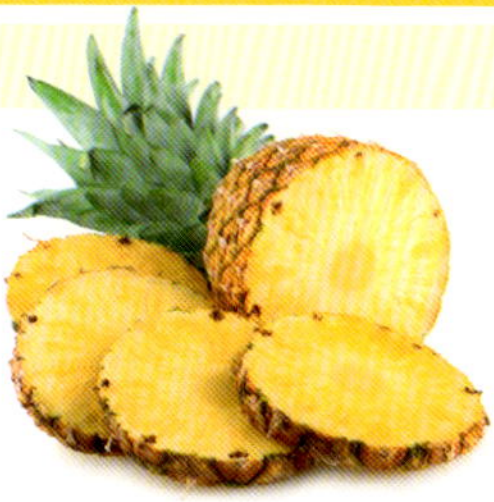

Description: The fruit acquired its name from its resemblance to a big pinecone. British Victorians loved this fragrant tropical plant, perhaps because it presented a challenge to cultivate in their cold climate. They expressed their admiration for the conic shape, chestnut-brown color, and stiff, spiny leaves by replicating pineapple imagery in wallpaper, drapery, upholstery, and other home decorations. A ripe pineapple has a sweet aroma and crisp, green leaves. Once on a trip to Maui, I visited a grocery store and sniffed the fruity aroma of really fresh pineapples as soon as I stepped inside. When you get pineapples ripe in the region where they are grown, they taste so much more juicy and delicious than the under-ripe, woody fruit we get at mainland supermarkets. Avoid specimens that smell slightly fermented, are discolored, marred by soft spots, or with brown-tinged leaves. Remove the crown and wash well before juicing.

Culinary Uses: Pineapples have been called nature's candy from the South Seas because they are so sweet. Pineapple juice substitutes reasonably well for table sugar in many recipes. To intensify the flavor, remove the crown and turn the pineapple upside down on a plate overnight to let the natural juices run down through the fruit. Lip-smacking delicious!

Nutrition: Because pineapples grow in the tropics near the sea, they contain a substantial amount of iodine. They also are renowned for their manganese content. The bromelian enzyme in the fruit, which is similar to the papain enzyme in papaya, breaks down protein. It is a digestive aid, dissolves blood clots, and cleans away dead tissue left over from surgery. Bromelian also helps strengthen muscles.

Lore: Pineapple is alleged to lift the spirits, bring back a departed lover, and purify and protect the body. Because it was a traditional home decoration for the wealthy, it has come to be associated with prosperity. In the *Language of Flowers* this fruit stands for "perfection." Add it to home blessing potions and formulas for monetary increase.

PLUM AND PRUNE

(Prunus domestica)

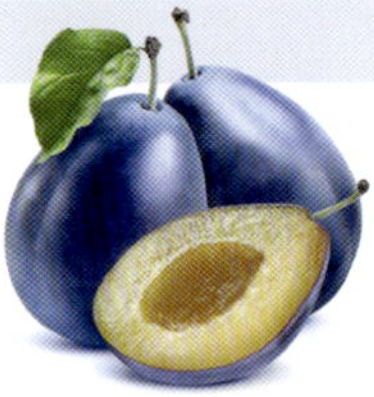

Description: Over 300 varieties of this relatively small, deciduous fruit tree of the rose family exist. The fruit is approximately the size of a medium tomato. Colors vary from green and yellow to purple, red, and blue. Damson plums are a favorite variety, and the one from which most American garden trees originate. Select plums with a sweet fragrance and good color that yield slightly to pressure. If necessary, ripen in a brown paper bag.

Culinary Uses: Prune whip and poached plums make delicious desserts, and plum wine is an Asian treat. Remember to remove the pit before juicing.

Nutrition: Like most fruit, plums contain many vitamins including A, C, and K, and beta-carotene as well as iron, and fiber. Beta carotene protects from lung and oral cavity cancers. Vitamin K may help retard the progression of Alzheimer's and facilitates bone metabolism and blood clotting.

Prunes are simply dried plums. Because they contain sorbitol and isatin, they are known for their laxative quality. Drinking plum juice (and plum wine!) helps immunize against heart disease and diabetes and cure cold sores. Caution: due to the presence of oxalic acid, people with urinary tract stones should avoid eating plums and prunes.

Lore: According to Welsh superstition, a plum that blooms in the December garden foretells that someone in the owner's home will die soon. In mythology, plums are associated with Saturn. This heavenly body is known as the planet of old age, so perhaps this is how the legend got started. The Chinese consider the plum to be a fruit of wisdom, and so the juice can be consumed in potions to improve general health, slow aging, and maybe turn you into a sage.

POMEGRANATE

(Punica granatum)

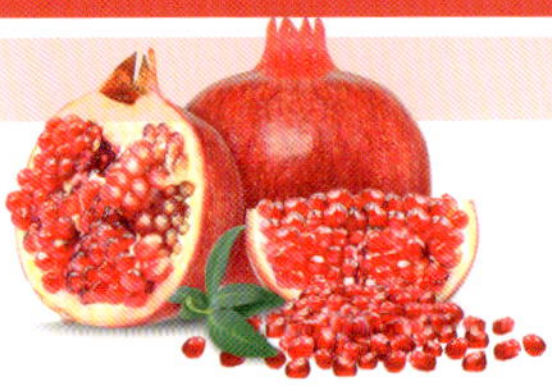

Description: This fruit is native to semitropical Asia and Persia. Even though pomegranates are as big as apples, botanically they are considered berries (as are tomatoes). The fruit grows on a thorny, deciduous bush that sports brilliant vermilion-colored flowers. They have hard, red skin that surrounds a juicy, translucent pulp and hundreds of edible, fleshy seeds. One gruesome bit of trivia is that the pomegranate gave its name to the grenade because of its shape and size and also because the grenade disperses fragments like the many seeds of the fruit.

Culinary Uses: Grenadine syrup is made from pomegranate juice. The juice can be reduced to a thick paste by boiling, and then added to meat dishes. Even though pomegranate juice recently has joined the ranks of the super health foods, I suggest you test before buying as you may not care for the taste. Pomegranate juice is often blended with other juices such as blueberry. Pomegranates are tricky to open. Use a sharp knife and make four cuts through the skin in the stem end. Work your way to the other side and remove the fruit. Even though the seeds are edible, I prefer to remove them and only juice the pulp. Sprinkle the dried seeds on sweet dishes and hummus.

Nutrition: Pomegranates are relatively high in calories—approximately one hundred per fruit. They include many nutrients such as calcium, copper, and vitamin K. This fruit helps prevent heart disorders and slows the growth of prostate and breast cancer. It also prevents cartilage deterioration in osteoarthritis and keeps LDL cholesterol from oxidizing to prevent atherosclerosis. Therefore, perhaps the ancient Babylonian belief that chewing the seeds would make them invincible may hold a kernel of truth.

Lore: This fruit is associated with the goddess Juno, who was much admired in biblical times. The Koran calls the pomegranate a gift from God. Some believe that the tree from which Eve ate the forbidden fruit in the Garden of Eden was actually a pomegranate, and not an apple. (Others believe it was the apricot.) On describing a beautiful woman, the *Song of Solomon* (4:3) relates that her cheeks are "like halves of a pomegranate behind your veil." In mythology, pomegranates are also sacred to Ceres, Persephone, Zeus, and Dionysus because their masses of seeds represent the bounty of the harvest. Drink pomegranate juice to help keep a secret or to have a secret wish granted. Also drink it whenever you want to bring fertility, prosperity, or renewal to your life.

POTATO

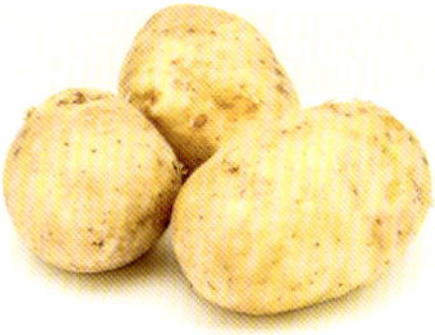

(Solanum tuberosum)

Description: Round or oblong potato tubers vary in color from white, to brown, red, and purple. They grow on a plant that originated high in the Andean region of South America.

Culinary Uses: This versatile vegetable can be boiled, baked, mashed, fried, creamed, chopped in potato salad or fruit, and even baked into bread. Peruvians claim that they have invented more than 200 recipes for potatoes. Having spent some time in that country, I can say that potatoes are a gourmet's delight in that region.

Nutrition: Potatoes are no higher in calories than most other vegetables. It is only the "calorific" toppings we add that makes them fattening. Potatoes contain some protein, are low in fat, and rich in healthy carbs to spur energy. In folk medicine, this vegetable has earned something of a reputation as a cure-all. Among its many virtues, it can be made into a plaster to alleviate inflammation from arthritis, hemorrhoids, abscesses, and sprains. The darker the color of the potato's flesh, the more vitamins it contains, with the purple variety being the most healthy. Unfortunately, the popular Idaho potato with its white flesh is the least healthy variety.

Lore: In the *Language of Flowers* potatoes mean "benevolence." In mythology this botanical is ruled by Saturn. Potatoes are consumed in potions for grounding as well as in formulas to improve health. They stand for safety, protection, and fulfillment.

PUMPKIN

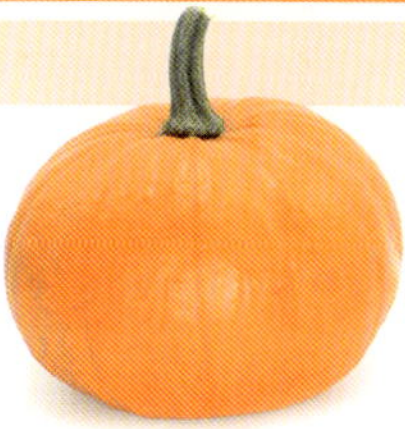

(Cucurbita pepo, C. mixta)

Description: The US produces over one billion pounds of pumpkins annually, most of which go to processing–not to make Halloween jack-o-lanterns. The big, round, furrowed, orange gourd grows on an annual vine that sports a prickly stem, tendrils, and round leaves. The same species includes other gourds such as acorn squash, zucchini, and straight neck. More than ninety percent of a pumpkin is water. The largest pumpkin ever grown weighed over 1,000 pounds, which means that an astounding 900 pounds of it was water.

Culinary Uses: Besides making pumpkin pie, this vegetable can be cooked in soups and puddings. The roasted, salted seeds provide a nourishing snack. Pumpkin pulp does not juice well, so you should blend it with milk or coconut milk if you are preparing a potion.

Nutrition: As you can tell by the orange color, pumpkins are loaded with beta-carotene, which converts to vitamin A in the body. They also contain a good portion of potassium (564 milligrams per cup) and unsaturated fats. Pumpkins are healthy for the kidneys and heart and help arrest the degenerative aspects of aging. They also tone the prostate and quell migraine headaches.

Lore: Like all gourds, pumpkins are associated with the moon, the heavenly body that symbolizes fertility and the bounty of the earth. Certainly the large size, round shape and numerous seeds evoke the idea of fecundity. In China pumpkins reign supreme in the plant world, where they are called "the emperor of vegetables." In the US at Halloween many people follow an age-old tradition of removing the pulp and carving their pumpkins into amusing or frightening faces. In former times, the candlelit pumpkins were meant to scare off evil spirits and the Devil. In the Cinderella fairy tale a pumpkin was transformed into the coach that transported her to the ball. Add pumpkin to potions for prosperity and better health and to help make dreams come true.

SPINACH

(Spinacea oleracea)

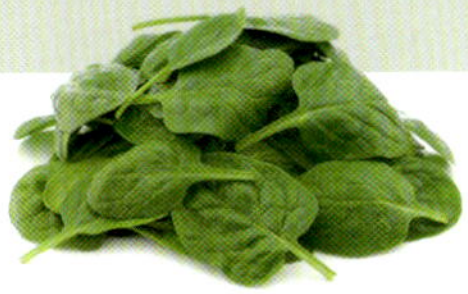

Description: Popeye's favorite vegetable is a leafy native of Persia and southwest Asia. Other plants that can be eaten like spinach include lamb's-quarters, watercress, mustard greens, dandelion leaves, and tea leaves. Choose bunches with dark green leaves that are crisp and firm. Like lettuce, this is a leafy, low-growing plant, so be sure to buy organic and wash the leaves well.

Culinary Uses: You might think that spinach in a smoothie potion is a bit farfetched, but I assure you it is not. Spinach juice combines harmoniously with carrot and celery. Moreover, a recent Dr. Oz show featured a breakfast smoothie that included spinach along with apple for sweetness (or mango, cooked sweet potato, or banana), cucumber, celery, parsley, lemon, and lime. Oz claims that it is his favorite breakfast drink.

Although the following anecdote does not represent a culinary recipe for spinach, it's certainly a nifty way to use this vegetable. The plant has been processed to form a film of chlorophyll, which produces electricity under the sun's rays. The energy is then stored for future use as electrical power. Now that's a way to take advantage of spinach energy that I bet Popeye never thought of!

Nutrition: Every child knows that the concentrated iron content of spinach makes you grow big and strong. It also contains an alphabet soup of vitamins and minerals, including A, B, C, E, K, phosphorous, and fiber. Spinach is considered a cancer inhibitor and may help prevent macular degeneration.

Lore: Add to potions for strength and vigor.

STRAWBERRY

(Fragraria ananassa, F. virginiana)

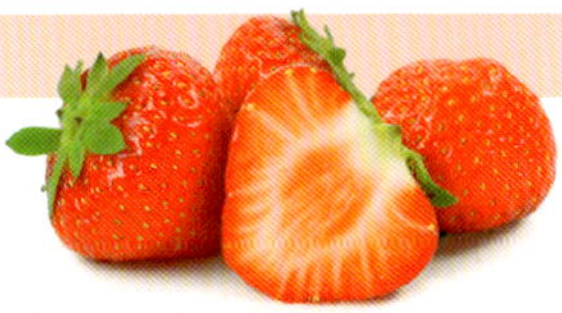

Description: The low-growing, red fruit of this leafy plant has been gathered in the wild by our ancestors for over 2,000 years. When colonists reached Virginia, they discovered that the local Native Americans had been cultivating strawberries practically forever. There is no skin on a strawberry, and the outside of the fruit is covered with hundreds of tiny seeds. Although strawberries grow in warm climates year round, they reach their peak in June and July.

Culinary Uses: The berry is a favorite jam and jelly and makes a sweet juice. Not to mention the delights of strawberries and cream!

Nutrition: Everyone knows the gastronomical pleasures of fat, juicy strawberries, but few realize that this plant was also a popular natural cosmetic ingredient in ancient times. Rather than spend a fortune on bleaching your teeth to remove yellow stains, try applying a combination of strawberry, raspberry and apple juice. Wait five minutes and clean off with bicarbonate of soda and warm water. Strawberries are an anti-abortive, astringent, diuretic, and laxative. The juice relieves sunburn pain, and the leaves in a beverage infusion make a fine female tonic.

Lore: In mythology, strawberries are associated with Venus, the Earth element, and the zodiac sign Libra. The leaves symbolize foresight. The loveliness of the leaves and fruit has inspired emblems for crests of the British gentry and crystal patterns as well as potions having to do with love, beauty, and fertility. The plump, red fruit inspired its *Language of Flowers* name, "perfect excellence." Folklore claims that fairies take delight in strawberry offerings.

The ambrosial scent of strawberry oil is said to draw good fortune when added to the bath. Drink the juice in potions to aid divination and clairvoyance.

TANGERINE

(Citrus nobilis var. deliciosa, C. reticulata)

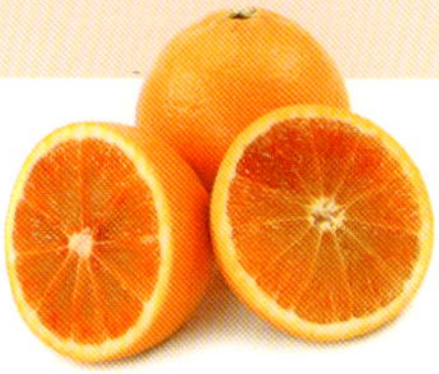

Description: Tangerines are a kind of orange, only smaller with looser skins that are easy to peel. The clementine, which is very small, but tender and sweet, is deep orange-colored. It is generally available during the winter holidays and therefore, makes a great stocking stuffer. The sweet Satsuma, honey mandarin, Minneola, and tangelo are other popular varieties. When selecting tangerines avoid loose, puffy skin or deep grooves, all of which indicate spoilage.

Culinary Uses: Besides juicing, try adding whole tangerine segments to fruit salads, or use the juice as an alternative to lemon in salad dressing.

Nutrition: The calcium in tangerines helps build strong teeth and healthy gums. Vitamins C and E are blood purifiers that expel toxins and remove excess water from the body. The vitamin B complex content is a super stress buster. Tangerine peel tea is good for lowering blood sugar levels, and the juice is a decongestant. Drink it to help banish yeast infections and intestinal parasites. Regular consumption of tangerines helps correct hormonal imbalances.

Lore: Tangerines were not introduced to Europe and America until Victorian times, and so they are late arrivals on the Western folklore scene. Nevertheless, a few legends can be found for this small, delicious fruit. For example, it is a favorite ingredient of sexual attraction potions. The oil, cold-pressed from the outer skin of the fruit, adds zest for life in potions. Both tangerine juice and cold-pressed oil will lend an exotic note to any potion. The juice is also said to harmonize the sacral chakra, probably because of its orange color.

TOMATO

(Lycopersicon esculentum)

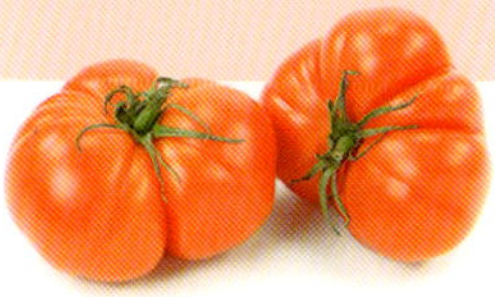

Description: At first, Europeans suspected this New World red, orange, or yellow vegetable (botanically, it is a berry!) of the nightshade family to be poisonous because other plants of the same family are fatal when consumed. Luckily, somebody took a chance on sampling them, and tomatoes have become staples in almost everybody's diet.

Many varieties exist, including the small plum tomatoes used in sauces, large beefsteak, and medium-sized slicers. They are usually round or globe-shaped. A few years ago, some horticulturalist got the bright idea to breed tomatoes into a square shape to make them easier to pack and ship. The idea went over with consumers like a square peg in a round hole. If you have a choice, go for organically grown tomatoes; they taste so much better than hothouse or commercially raised ones.

Culinary Uses: Juicy tomatoes combine well with carrots, celery, and parsley in juice. They form the base for a variety of soups and sauces, and of course, can be pureed or used as a paste. A popular tomato-cucumber-based soup is Spanish gazpacho.

Nutrition: Tomatoes help close festering wounds and flush toxins from the liver.

Lore: Once Europeans overcame their suspicion of the tomato, they decided it made an excellent aphrodisiac, and nicknamed the plant the "love apple." It was once considered a candidate for the "elixir of life," reputed to regenerate life, guard good health, and bring prosperity to the home. Superstition dictates that if you place a large, red tomato on your kitchen windowsill, it will keep evil spirits at bay. Include tomatoes in love, prosperity, better health, and home blessing potions.

VANILLA

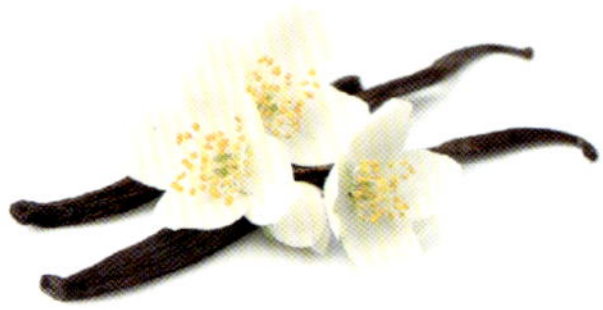

(Latin Name: Vanilla planifolia, V. tahitensis)

Description: The seductive flavor of vanilla originates in the pod (known as a bean) of a greenish-yellow creeping orchid native to Mexico and Central America. These days Tahiti produces some of the best gourmet vanilla.

Culinary Uses: Vanilla bean and vanilla extract enjoy an honored place in most kitchens. Vanilla lends a voluptuous, sweet flavor to liquid potions such as liqueurs, teas, smoothies, and herbal infusions, and it is also used widely in baking. Often it is coupled with almond extract to enhance each other's flavor. Don't faint when you go to buy a vanilla bean and see how expensive it is. You can reuse it many times in cooking as long as you wash and dry it after each use.

Nutrition: Vanilla is considered a sexual stimulant. At the same time, the B-complex vitamins it contains have a calming effect. Add the extract to potions to neutralize the little frustrations and contretemps of daily life. The very scent of vanilla helps regulate the nervous system as well as the metabolism. The flavor combines well with black tea as well as with blueberry, clove, cranberry, honey, honeybush, and pomegranate infusions.

Lore: Vanilla is the premier go-to ingredient for Voodoo love potions, at least according to nineteenth century New Orleans Voodoo queen, Marie Laveau.

YAM AND SWEET POTATO

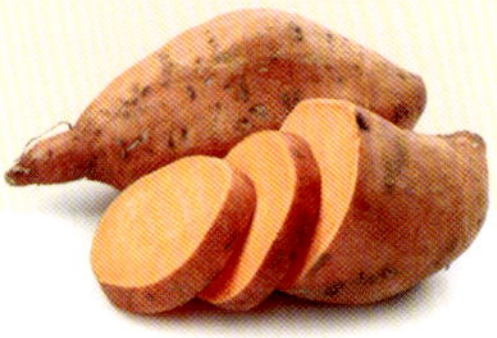

Dioscorea alata (Yam), Ipomoea batatas (Latin for sweet potato, but it is actually a plant of the morning glory family)

Description: These moist-fleshed tubers from different botanical species taste much the same and are used interchangeably in potion-crafting.

Culinary Uses: The flavor combines well with carrots and beets. Because they are so fibrous, I suggest you combine the roots with a juicier vegetable or with milk when blending. Often they are eaten baked, like potatoes, chopped, cooked, or candied.

Nutrition: In spite of the fact that these two vegetables look and taste similar, they possess different nutrients. Sweet potatoes have more vitamins A and E, calcium, and iron, and are anti-inflammatory. Yams can exacerbate inflammation, but they contain more omega-3 fatty acids and help remove heavy metals from the body.

Lore: These tubers stand for charity, compassion, and the earth's bounty. Consume them in potions for fertility and creativity.

Appendix B

TWELVE TERRIFIC TISANE HERBS

So many enchanting herbs and so little space to write about them! It was hard to make choices, but finally I whittled down my list to twelve healthy, flavorful botanicals that are also useful in potion-crafting. Prepare them as singles or blend some together according to your needs and creativity. To impart zing add bits of the spices described in Chapter 6.

ALFALFA LEAF

(Medicago sativa)

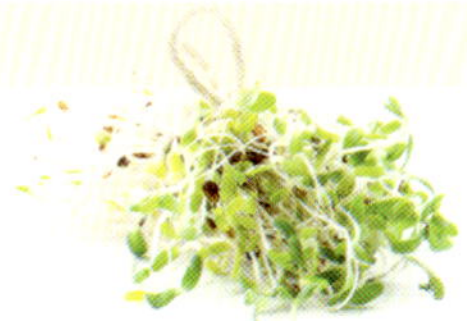

If you live nearby or pass through agricultural fields, you've probably seen alfalfa growing. This grassy perennial has been fed to horses for centuries because it has a high vitamin and mineral content. In fact, our word for this grass originates in Arabic, where its common name means "father of all foods." Alfalfa is as good for humans as it is for equines. The blades contain plenty of vitamins A, B, C, and K; organic salts; essential enzymes, and the minerals calcium, magnesium, phosphorous, and potassium.

This herb tastes grassy like green tea and looks yellow in the cup, so it can represent this hue in color healing. Drink the infusion to recover fast from an illness, lower your blood pressure, and help stop hemorrhaging. Because of its many nutrients, alfalfa can go a long way toward replacing lost vitamins and minerals when a person is dieting to lose weight. To enhance alfalfa's flavor, blend it with perkier botanicals like lemon balm, red clover, or spearmint.

ANGELICA

(Angelica archangelica)

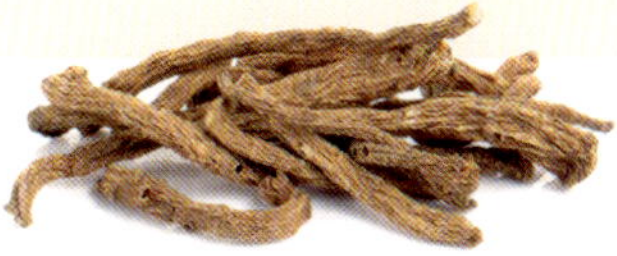

This thick-stemmed, leafy plant of the carrot family flourishes in cool climates. Use the roots, leaves, and seeds in infusions. Angelica tastes best when blended with lemony herbs like verbena and balm, minty herbs, or red clover. The seeds ground and brewed in an infusion relieve gas pains. They are also the signature ingredient of Chartreuse liqueur. Angelica is a diuretic and tonic for the stomach and intestines. Drink the celery-flavored infusion as an alternative to cranberry juice to alleviate the symptoms of a urinary tract infection. Since it is also a stimulant, any part of the plant can be brewed in a tisane to uplift body and spirit.

Legend has it that angelica was revealed to humanity by Archangel Michael as a remedy against contagious diseases, poison, and plague. Some people use angelica as a sprinkling tea inside the home to protect from evildoers. In the *Language of Flowers* this plant symbolizes "inspiration."

BLUEBERRY LEAF AND FRUIT

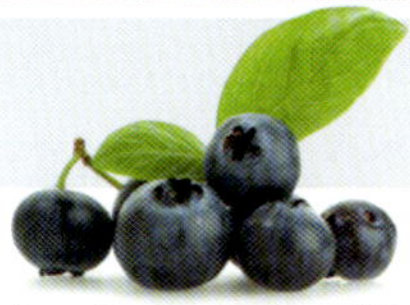

(Vaccinium corymbosum Highbush Blueberry)
(V. cyanococcus American Blueberry)

The native North American blueberry plant has thrived in the wild for thousands of years, but has only been under cultivation commercially since the beginning of the twentieth century. Blueberry juice tastes mild on its own, and combines successfully with the juices of apples, pears, and pineapples. It also makes a delicious liqueur. The part of the plant generally used to make a tisane is the leaf, but it never hurts to squirt in some blueberry juice to sweeten and fortify your brew.

Over the past few years, blueberry fruit and leaf have gained the reputation as a super food–not for no good reason. Both berries and leaves are rich in fiber, vitamins C, B-6, and K, manganese, and anthocyanin, the antioxidant that helps keep cancer-causing free radicals at bay. The skins also contain resveratrol, which like red grapes, has a positive effect on the heart. The berries and leaves, which are the part consumed as a tisane, help lessen cognitive decline in the elderly, lower blood pressure, prevent urinary tract infections, and mitigate symptoms of neurological diseases. While the berries contain a lot of sugar, the tea made from the leaves can lower a diabetic's need for insulin. In folklore, this plant belongs to the planet Venus, so it is also added to potions for fertility and prosperity.

CHAMOMILE FLOWER

(Matricaria recutita)

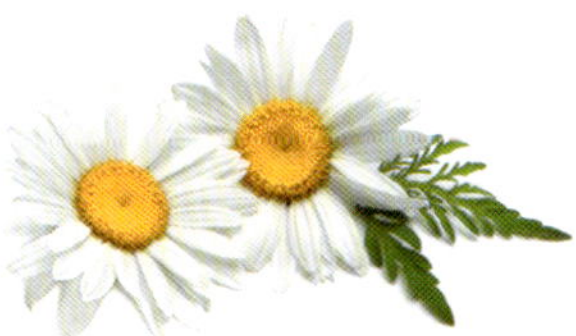

The apple-scented flowers of this low-growing spreader look like daisies. Several varieties exist including German (good in an infusion), Hungarian (bitter-tasting), Roman (the showy flowers are not edible, but are used in potpourris), and Egyptian (usually the cheapest.) I make a hair rinse from the dried blossoms to add highlights to my blond curls. Brewed chamomile looks yellow in the cup and so can represent that hue in color healing. However, the extract, which can also be consumed by the drop, is bright blue. Add a couple of drops of the essence to a glass of spring water for a blue-hued healing potion. Because chamomile tea is a mild sedative, it is a time-honored aid to promote a restful sleep and ease a troubled mind. It also makes a great digestive tonic.

In potion-crafting, the tisane is drunk or used as a sprinkling tea to increase business and draw wealth, especially if you rinse your hands in the liquid before beginning the business day.

Serves according to amounts prepared

Sleep Tight

Ingredients

Combine equal parts: Chamomile, Lemon balm, Rose petals, Rose hips

¼ part valerian root, cut

¼ part dried orange peel

Directions

Use one-half teaspoon per cup and drink at bedtime.

DANDELION LEAF AND ROOT

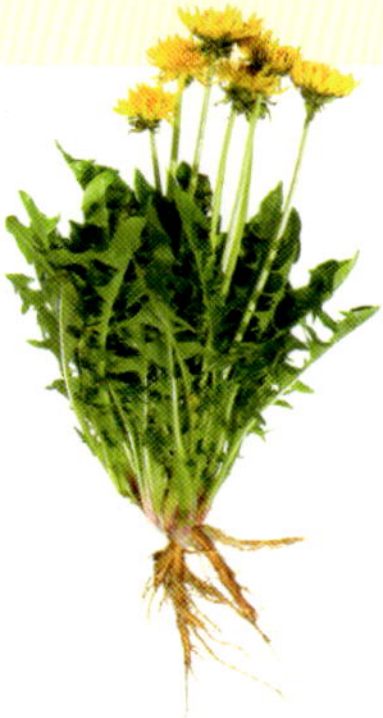

(Taraxacum officinale)

Fresh, young dandelion leaves make crispy additions to springtime salads. Both the leaves and root go into preparing tisanes, although each tastes quite different. Both parts contain large amounts of vitamin C. Herbalists recommend this botanical to help dissolve kidney stones and cure urinary and kidney infections. Roasted dandelion root, which contains no caffeine, is sometimes substituted for coffee, especially when combined with chicory. Naturopathic healers prescribe it to help overcome an emotionally traumatic event.

It's likely that most dandelions you run across thrive in lawns and parks. Make sure they haven't been sprayed with pesticides or chemical fertilizers before picking them. To be perfectly safe I recommend you buy your dandelion leaf and root at an herb store or natural grocers.

HIBISCUS FLOWER

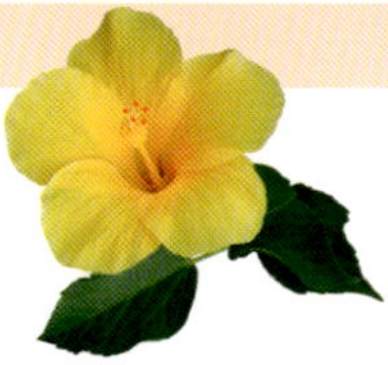

(Hibiscus rosa-sinensis)

You may recognize hibiscus flowers because the plant is a foundation shrub ubiquitous in gardens worldwide. The lovely, large purple, white, red, pink, or orange blossoms are the part used to make infusions. In Egypt, hibiscus flowers comprise the main ingredient of the liquid refreshment known as Karkade.

As you learned from the hibiscus water recipe in Chapter 1, the flowers turn red when boiled, and therefore represent that hue in color healing. The liquid is also sweet enough to be used as a sugar substitute in potions, although it also tastes somewhat astringent.

Hibiscus is an anti-inflammatory that also helps increase circulation, but at the same time can lower blood pressure. The tisane is a diuretic and appetite suppressant, which makes it a fond choice for dieters. In the *Language of Flowers* hibiscus stands for "delicate beauty," and is a prime ingredient of love potions.

LAVENDER LEAF AND FLOWER

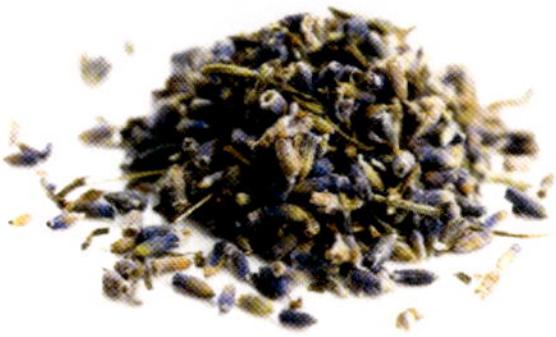

(Lavandula vera, L. angustifolia, L. spica)

The spiky flowers and leaves of this shrubby perennial make a fresh, clean, sweetly aromatic addition to teas and herbal infusions. The taste is enhanced by combining it with flowery elements such as rose or mild, citrusy flavors that you find in tangerine or lemon balm.

As to its virtues, some herbalists consider lavender to be something of a cure-all. It is a metabolic and respiratory stimulant and tonic for the central nervous system. Herbalists prescribe it for nervous exhaustion, headache, migraine, and depression. This botanical has been used in folk medicine as an antispasmodic for bronchitis, vomiting, and colic. Some claim it is also effective against typhoid fever, diphtheria, black widow and some snake bites, stings, skin lesions, asthma, insomnia, and bad breath. The essence helps regenerate skin cells and slows the wrinkling process. Lavender's stimulating action can help promote quick delivery of a baby by increasing contractions as well as ease common muscular aches and pains.

Probably because of its clean flavor, lavender infusions are sometimes drunk in purification rites. This herb is said to heighten awareness and prepare the psyche to receive the spirit by grounding and centering. It makes an excellent infusion to accompany meditation.

LEMON BALM LEAF

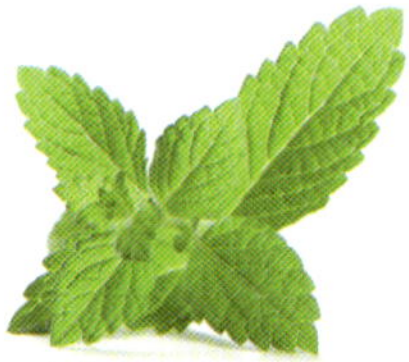

(Melissa officinalis)

The lemony-tasting leaves of this perennial are one of my favorite additions to any kind of iced tea. When I use them as a single ingredient, I boil the leaves and let them cool before adding ice. Lemon balm is good for the health, too. Drink the infusion of the leaf to ease a sore throat, lower your temperature and soothe aching teeth from sinus infection. Lemon balm also has a gentle stimulant and tonic action. Apply it externally to ease the itch from bee stings.

While lemon balm comprises a popular ingredient of love potions, I think this botanical is at its best when taken as a tisane to help speakers organize their thoughts before lecturing in public. Some herbalists recommend steeping the leaves in wine and drinking the brew to chase away melancholy and rejuvenate body, mind, and spirit. I'm not so sure, however, that the happy feelings don't come from the wine rather than the herb.

NETTLE LEAF

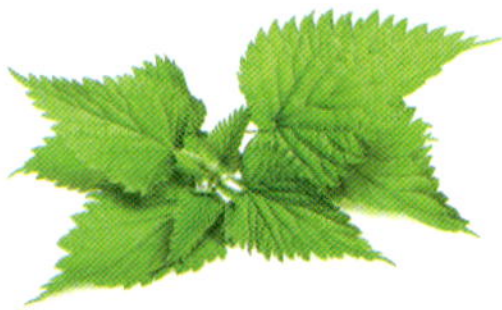

(Urtica dioica)

The blame goes to the Romans for first sowing in Britain this plant, now so difficult to eradicate. Legend has it that they did it to rub the prickly leaves on their bodies to improve their circulation in what they thought was an unbearably cold climate. This scourge of the English countryside is perfectly harmless once the leaves dry. In fact, the nettle is an important ingredient in medicinal infusions. The leaves are a blood purifier that treat anemia and help the body absorb nutrients. They also strengthen the uterus and entire female reproductive system. Nettles have also been used to manage asthma symptoms and help with weight loss. Since they are so prickly, some herbalists claim that, by analogy nettles help relieve uncomfortable situations and halt jealous rumors. In folklore, ancient Nordic people used to throw nettles on the fire during a thunderstorm in the belief that they kept people safe from Thor's lightning bolts.

PEPPERMINT LEAF

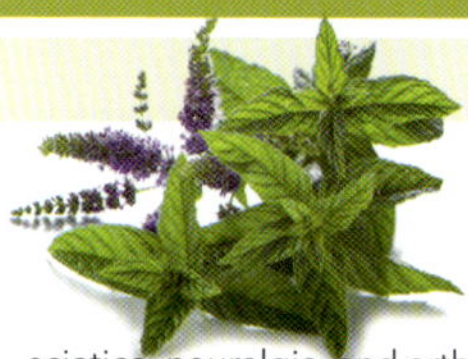

(Mentha piperita)

This is probably the best known of all the mints, and the one with the strongest flavor. The herb thrives in just about any shady, damp place and is almost impossible to eradicate once it takes hold in the garden. The leaves are an anti-inflammatory and a pain killer in cases of sciatica, neuralgia, and arthritis. It is also a decongestant, digestive, antiseptic against infectious diseases, and calmative for headaches and migraines. Small amounts of a decoction of peppermint oil on the skin help eliminate herpes, ringworm, poison ivy, eczema, dermatitis, and scabies. Peppermint is known to stop milk flow, so it should not be used by nursing mothers. Peppermint has a strong flavor in an infusion. Other mints you might try and which taste milder include bergamot, chocolate mint, curly mint, orange mint, and spearmint.

Peppermint is alleged to draw love and excitement, cement partnerships, and improve the memory. Use it in potions to heal the Earth. Pluto–the former planet, not the dog!–is said to have changed his wife's rival Mentha into a peppermint plant; so, in the *Language of Flowers* this Plutonian herb refers to both the "coldness of fear" and the "warmth of love." A drop of the essence will brighten any potion. If drunk before bedtime, peppermint tea is said to encourage prophetic dreams. I've tried this, and although my dreams were vivid, so far none have been prophetic. Peppermint tisanes also are thought to attract good luck, happiness, and foster new beginnings.

RASPBERRY LEAF AND FRUIT

(Rubus idaeus)

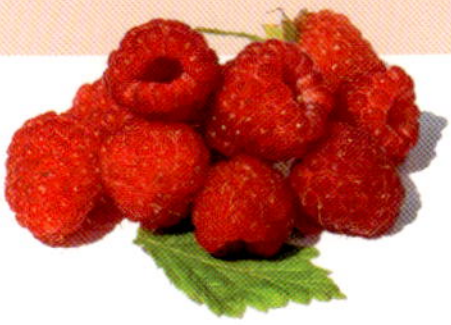

Raspberries are a delicious sweet red or black fruit that grow on prickly bushes, usually near a water source. Herbalists call the raspberry leaf "the pregnancy herb" because it is an astringent and antispasmodic that strengthens the uterus. An infusion of the leaves is also drunk to lessen menstrual cramps, calm an upset stomach, lessen a fever, and eliminate canker sores. Raspberries will sweeten any potion, as the next recipe shows.

Give That Cold a RASPBERRY TISANE

Serves 2

Nothing is more unwelcome than a cold that hangs on. Get rid of it for good with the following hot beverage infusion.

Ingredients

- 2 teaspoons raspberry leaves
- 1 teaspoon raspberry juice, or puree
- 1 teaspoon elder flowers
- ½ teaspoon fresh lemon peel, grated
- ½ teaspoon fresh ginger root, grated

Directions

Brew an infusion from the ingredients and enjoy.

ROSE PETAL AND HIP

(Rosa genus)

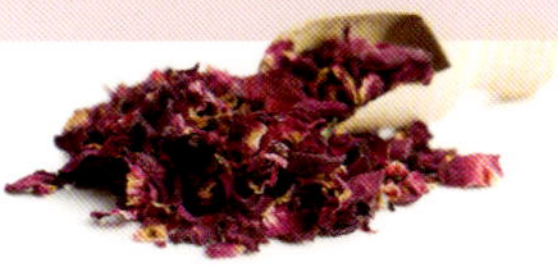

The rose is probably the most universally recognized and beloved flower throughout the world. Rose hips (the mature seed head) are very sweet and contain large amounts of vitamin C. The flower petals make a lovely edible garnish and exude a light, delicate aroma in teas and tisanes. Rose petals are an astringent and stomachic.

In several religions, the rose is an emblem of high aspiration. Rosebuds, besides being the name of Citizen Kane's childhood sled, symbolize love and devotion. Rose hips, buds, and flowers make pretty tisanes.

Here is a recipe that takes full advantage of both the petals and the hips. This infusion is loaded with vitamin C. Use only dry ingredients so you can store the leftovers. Mix them together well and place in a big, wide-mouthed jar.

Glossary

This glossary is divided into two parts. The first section defines general vocabulary and the second section is dedicated to medical terms used in this book.

General Terms

Annual: A plant that completes its entire life cycle from seed to growth to seed during one growing season, after which it dies to the ground completely. Some annuals are perennials in warm climates. Examples: cucumber, dill.

Agua Frescas: Fruit-based, non-carbonated, sweetened waters hailing from Mexico. These beverages substitute for sodas and are often drunk at mealtime.

Aperitif: A French loan word used to describe an alcoholic drink taken before meals to stimulate the appetite.

Biennial: A plant that takes two seasons to complete its entire life cycle, usually producing flowers and seeds during the second year. Example: celery.

Camellia sinensis: Latin name for the tea bush, also known as *Thea sinensis camellia*.

Chicha Morada: A nonalcoholic juice of Peruvian origin made, in part, from purple corn.

Chocolate: A food preparation made from the roasted, husked, and ground seeds of the *Theobroma* cacao tree. The seeds, known as beans, are roasted and ground, and often sweetened and flavored with vanilla and fruits, nuts, and/or spices such as cinnamon. Milk chocolate is produced by adding milk powder.

Cocoa: To make cocoa from the cocoa bean the producer powders the bean and removes the butter fat. Therefore, cocoa is considered healthier than chocolate.

Cooler: A refreshing drink served cold.

Cordial: A refreshing drink especially designed to stimulate the heart and revive the spirits. Often it contains alcohol.

Cut and Sifted (acronym: c/s): Process by which a botanical is chopped into ¼- to ½-inch pieces, the smallest particles are sifted away, and the plant is dried. The result eliminates most of the powder and retains the desired part of the plant for culinary and medicinal use.

Element: One of the four primary substances which ancient cultures believed engendered life. Western civilizations name four elements earth, fire, air, and water. Most Asian cultures name five–earth, fire, metal, wood, water.

Elixir: In cooking and herbal medicine, a sweetened liquid that contains alcohol.

Ethnic Pot: Anointed spout at the rim. It is also called an *Ibrik*.

Extract: In both cooking and herbal medicine, a plant preparation of a liquid or viscous consistency containing one or more botanical substances.

Herb: Any botanical that dies down completely during the winter in cold climates, whose leaves, seeds, roots, or flowers are used for flavoring, food, medicine, and/or perfume. Example: thyme.

Infusion: A method of brewing tea or an herbal beverage by pouring boiling water over leaves, flowers, and/or small stems of a plant, and allowing the liquid to steep for from two-to-ten minutes. Under five minutes of brewing time works best for beverage drinks; more than that and you get a medicinal infusion.

Inquirer: In divination, the person making the inquiry; that is, the one having a coffee-ground or tea leaf reading, or any kind of intuitive reading; sometimes referred to as the "querent" or "client."

Juice: Liquid derived from a single ingredient or combination of fruits and/or vegetables. Since another meaning for this term is "the essence of something," a juice can be thought of as containing the essence of the fruit or vegetable.

Julep: A syrup (defined below) mixed with water, whiskey, or brandy, and meant for immediate consumption. Juleps are often concocted using herbs, with mint juleps probably being the most popular.

Language of Flowers: A book containing symbolic meanings for plants taken from folklore, mythology, art, and literature.

Malt: Barley or other grain that is steeped in water until it germinates, and then is dried in a kiln. Malt is used in brewing some alcoholic drinks such as beer and ale. In powdered form, it can be added to milk, ice cream, or yogurt to create a thick shake.

Ochazuke Soup: A hot soup of Japanese origin made from a green tea base.

Perennial: A plant that grows and produces flowers and seed for many seasons, whether or not it dies to the ground in winter. Examples: peppermint, apple.

PETE, PET: Acronyms for polyethylene terephthalate. This strong and stiff member of the polyester family of polymers can be spun into fibers or blow-molded into disposable beverage containers. Sometimes they leak carcinogens into the liquid contained in the bottle. Apple juice is especially susceptible.

Philter (also spelled Philtre): A mystical drink that aims to produce certain sentiments or sensations.

Potion: From Latin *potare,* meaning "to drink." A potion is a liquid drunk in the belief that it will produce a special effect. Potions are meant to invoke various forms of spiritual energy such as protection, strength, or universal love. The term also refers to liquid substances with magical properties that are not for internal consumption. However, such drinks are not the focus of this book.

Punch: A drink sweetened and flavored with fruit juices, spices, and often with wine or liquor.

Sauce: A liquid or soft dressing mixed with or poured over food to improve the flavor. Sauces can be used as toppings for cakes, custards, fruit, and ice cream as well as for savory dishes. Example: béchamel sauce.

Shake: A cold drink made from milk and flavoring and blended or shaken with ice and/or ice cream or yogurt until it turns frothy.

Smoothie: A thick, smooth cold drink concocted from fresh pureed fruit blended with ice, ice cream, yogurt, or milk, and sometimes with the addition of protein or other vitamin supplements. Brazilian *vitaminas* (see definition below) represent a type of smoothie. Smoothie mixes and starter bases are also available.

Soup: A liquid dish prepared by cooking vegetables, fish, poultry, and/or meat in water, milk, fruit, or vegetable juices. Soups may be drunk hot or cold, and are often served as the first course of a main meal. Examples: mushroom soup (hot), gazpacho (cold).

Sprinkling Tea: An infusion made from botanicals, which may or may not include tea leaves, and water with the intention of dispersing it around a room, on clothing, inside a vehicle, etc. Sprinkling teas are not meant to be consumed.

Stevia (Stevia rebaudiana)

A substance extracted from a native Paraguayan herb that is many times sweeter than sugar, but is calorie-free. Also known as sweet leaf, it is used to sweeten food and drinks.

Syrup: A sweet remedy for cough or sore throat. An advantage of syrup is that it retards the deterioration rates of sensitive herbs. To make a syrup, mix two ounces or so of the herb required in one part water or fruit juice, then boil, strain, and add two ounces of honey.

Tea: A beverage or sprinkling infusion made from the leaves of the *Camellia sinensis* tree. Herbal tea is a popular name for an infusion made from other botanicals. To be perfectly accurate, they are not proper teas, but tisanes or herbal infusions.

Tisane: A drinking infusion made from botanicals other than the tea plant, popularly referred to as an herbal tea or infusion.

Turkish Coffee: Also known as Greek coffee, it is a fine, powdery coffee usually blended with sugar and spices, and often used in coffee-ground reading.

Vitaminas: A Brazilian beverage drunk cold and lauded for its healthy attributes, hence the name. *Vitaminas* are a kind of smoothie that mixes fruit juices and/or milk, sugar, and ice, often with the addition of oats, and is processed in a blender. *Vitaminas* bars have been popular in Brazil long before the introduction of the smoothie to the US consumer.

Medical Terms

ADD: Acronym for Attention Deficit Disorder, a disease, often diagnosed in childhood, which manifests in a pattern of symptoms that may include a short attention span, hyperactivity, impulsive behavior, and occupational and social interference.

Alzheimer's Disease: A form of dementia caused by degeneration and destruction of brain cells and characterized by memory loss, inability to perform daily tasks, and/or aggressive behavior.

Anthocyanin, cyanin: Blue, violet, and red pigments found in plants such as rose petals and cornflowers, which may deter diabetes and breast cancer and keep arteries free from obstructions.

Antibacterial: A substance that checks the growth and/or effects of toxic bacteria (one-cell organisms that contain no chlorophyll and some of which can cause disease).

Antibiotic: A substance that literally kills life by inhibiting the growth of or destroying harmful bacteria, amoebas and, according to some sources, even some viruses. Antibiotics also stimulate the body's defense mechanisms.

Antihistamine: A substance that minimizes the action of histamines; that is, symptoms of allergic conditions such as hay fever.

Anti-inflammatory: An agent that reduces swelling, heat, and pain associated with inflammations.

Antioxidant: A substance that removes potentially damaging oxidizing agents in the blood. Examples include vitamins C and E.

Antiseptic: An agent applied to the skin to destroy or prevent bacterial growth, sepsis, and putrefaction. If the matter is herbal, it will prevent new growth only.

Antispasmodic: A substance that prevents or diminishes muscle spasms, cramps, convulsions, and nervous tension.

Aphrodisiac: A tonic to improve sexual potency and power.

Aromatherapy: A technique by which essential oils are ingested, applied externally to the skin, or inhaled in order to heal body, emotions, mind, and spirit.

Aromatic: A substance that exudes a fragrant, spicy odor and is used to make other drugs and potions taste better.

Astringent: Something that constricts and binds soft tissue. Astringents are used to check internal and external secretions like diarrhea and bleeding.

Blood Purifier: A term used in herbal medicine to describe a detoxifying agent that neutralizes acidity in the blood.

Caffeine: A stimulant present in tea, coffee, cocoa, and some other botanicals that can aggravate high blood pressure, overstimulate the heart, and cause breakouts in those with acne-prone skin.

Carcinogen: A substance that tends to produce cancer.

Carminative: A substance that relieves flatulence.

Carotenoid: An antioxidant present in red, yellow, and orange fruit and vegetables that easily converts to vitamin A in the body.

Catechin: A type of flavonoid (described below) considered more powerfully antioxidant than vitamins A, C, E, and beta-carotene.

Chakra: In various Eastern religions and health systems, a point of spiritual energy that exists in the etheric matter outside the body. Hinduism and Buddhism identify seven traditional chakras; the Western system of Ceremonial Magick identifies five.

Chlorophyll: A green substance present in plants that interacts with the sun's energy, carbon dioxide, and water to infuse them with a green color. Chlorophyll aids digestion in the human body and helps mitigate bad breath.

Cholesterol: A waxy, fatty substance produced in the liver and found in all parts of the body that harmonizes vitamin D and digestion. High Density Lipoprotein (HDL) cholesterol is considered "good" because it moves cholesterol from the tissues to the liver. On the other hand, Low Density Lipoprotein (LDL) cholesterol moves cholesterol into the tissues, including the arteries, which can cause them to clog.

Decoction: A strong tea prepared for medicinal purposes. It is usually made from roots, barks, and/or large seeds of plants and must be simmered or steeped for at least fifteen to twenty minutes, then strained before drinking. These highly concentrated teas usually do not have a pleasant taste.

Decongestant: A treatment or medication that relieves stuffiness of the nasal passages and/or the bronchial tubes.

Diabetes: A disease caused by high blood sugar and characterized by excessive urination.

Diuretic: A urinary tonic that increases the flow of urine when taken as an infusion.

Doctrine of Signatures: A theory of medicine developed during the Middle Ages to treat disease. Among other things, the doctrine stated that botanicals that looked like body parts were linked to them and could be used to treat and cure diseases of those organs. For example, the eyebright flowers that resembled eyes could be distilled to cure eye diseases. Bladderwrack, a seaweed that looks something like little human bladders, could be consumed to treat diseases of the bladder. Colors and odors were also associated in the same way.

EGCG: An acronym for epigallocatechin-3-gallate, a flavonoid present in green tea and some fruit and vegetables that may help boost the immune system and keep free radicals from damaging and destroying body cells.

Electrolyte: Certain salts and minerals that conduct electrical impulses through the body and which enable muscle contraction, contribute to flexibility and balance, and infuse the system with energy.

Emollient: A dressing, cream, or ointment that soothes, softens, and protects the skin.

Expectorant: A medicine that expels mucus from the respiratory tract by promoting coughing.

Flatulence: Gas passed from the stomach and intestines, commonly known as farting.

Flavonoid (also called a bioflavonoid): A plant-based nutrient and antioxidant that can fight various cancers and heart disease. Flavonoids are present in certain botanicals, including tea, fruit, and vegetables.

Free Radicals: Incomplete molecules in the body that attach themselves to healthy cells and tissues and can rob them of oxygen, causing their deterioration and death.

Herbal Medicine: The study and use of medicinal botanicals derived from natural plant substances to treat and prevent disease.

Homeopathy: A system of medicine based on the aspect of the theory of the Doctrine of Signatures, where it is believed that "like cures like." Minute doses of substances are given to the patient, which in a healthy person would cause symptoms of the disease.

Laxative: Something that acts gently to promote bowel movements.

Metabolism: A chemical and physical process of food assimilation.

Narcotic: An agent that diminishes the action of the nervous and muscular systems, lessens pain, and induces sleep, stupor, and insensibility.

Nervine: Also called a nerve tonic, it is a preparation designed to release nervous tension and irritability and nourish the nervous system. Nervines restore the balance of energy within the body.

Oxalic Acid: A substance found in fruit and vegetables such as rhubarb, sorrel, and spinach, which in large doses can inhibit the assimilation of calcium and iron in the body.

Parkinson's disease: A chronic and progressive disease that affects muscle coordination and movement. It can be characterized by involuntary tremors, slow movement, muscle stiffness, and impaired balance and coordination. Celebrities afflicted by the disease have included Katharine Hepburn, Linda Ronstadt, and Michael J. Fox.

Pectin: A water soluble sugar acid present in many fruits including apple, grapefruit, and plum.

pH: A measure of acidity or alkalinity in a solution such as water.

Phytochemical: Chemicals naturally found in fruit, vegetables, and nuts, which can have a positive impact on health. Examples include carotenoids, lutein, lycopene, flavonoids, and beta carotene.

PMS: Acronym for Pre-Menstrual Syndrome, a condition that may occur in women two to ten days before onset of menstruation that is characterized by breast tenderness, abdominal bloating, irritability, headache, fatigue, and/or depression.

Preservative: A substance with the ability to retard rotting or spoilage.

Psoriasis: A skin condition characterized by redness, flaking, and irritation.

Resveratrol: An antioxidant and anti-inflammatory present in plants such as grapes and mulberries that has a positive effect on the cardiovascular system and may help promote weight loss.

Second Potting: A method for reducing the amount of caffeine in tea by brewing a pot of leaves, discarding the water, and using the brewed leaves to make another potful.

Sedative: A remedy to quiet the central nervous system and induce sleep. If it also soothes pain, it is called an "anodyne."

Shingles: A painful inflammation of nerve ganglia, generally forming rash and blisters around the middle of the body. Shingles are caused by a reactivation of the chickenpox virus.

Silicon: An essential trace mineral important for bone, joint, and skin health that tends to diminish with age. Bananas, beer, string beans, and most water contain silicon.

Stimulant: An agent that increases the body's circulation and breaks up obstructions that reduce the body's energy reserves, such as prolonged, low-grade fevers or sluggish digestion. Stimulants warm the body by increasing metabolism and encourage the system to throw off illness. Not recommended in cases of nervousness, hypertension, ulcerative colitis, or when the body is extremely weak from disease.

Tannins: Astringent polyphenol compounds that are present in many plants, including the *Camellia sinensis* and coffee trees. The tannins in tea and coffee are similar to the substances in red wine. They interact with the proteins in the mouth to give tea, coffee, and some other botanicals their color, astringency and flavor.

Theobromine and Theophylline: Crystalline alkaloids present in the cacao bean, cola nut, and tea that act as a diuretic and heart stimulant, and which also relax the muscles and bronchial passages to reduce stress.

Tonic: A preparation that promotes the functioning of the body's systems, maintains health, and increases energy. It is ingested as a preventative when no disease is present.

Toxin: An unstable, poisonous compound that can cause certain diseases.

Tranquilizer: Something that induces a serene mental state free from anxiety and agitation.

Triglyceride: A type of lipid found in the blood. When you eat, that which your body does not require for immediate energy use is stored as triglycerides in the fat cells for later use. If you overeat, the triglycerides build up and can lead to atherosclerosis, heart disease, and stroke.

Bibliography

Books

Anon. *El YerbaLibro*. (Santa Ana, CA: Calli Casa Editorial, 1997.)

Anon. *Everyday Witchcraft*. (New York, NY: Dell, 1972.)

Anon. *The Ancient Book of Formulas*. (Dallas, TX: Dorene, 1967.)

Barash, Cathy Wilkinson. *Edible Flowers from Garden to Palate*. (Golden, CO: Fulcrum, 1993.)

Bethel, May. *The Healing Power of Herbs*. (London, England: Thorsons, 1968.)

Beyerl, Paul. *The Master Book of Herbalism*. (Custer, WA: Phoenix, 1984.)

Bias, Clifford. *Ritual Book of Magic*. (York Beach, ME: Samuel Weiser, 1982 rpt. 1981.)

Birren, Faber. *Color Psychology and Color Therapy: A Factual Study of the Influence of Color on Human Life*. (Secaucus, NJ: Citadel Press, 1961 rpt. 1950.)

Blofeld, John. *The Chinese Art of Tea*. (Boston, MA: Shambhala Publications, 1985.)

Borino, Bob. *Herbal Remedies*. (West Palm Beach, FL: Globe Communications, 1983.)

Calbom, Cherie, and Maureen Keane. *Juicing for Life: A Guide to the Health Benefits of Fresh Fruit and Vegetable Juicing*. (Garden City Park, NY: Avery Publishing Group, 1992.)

Chamberlain, Mary. *Old Wives' Tales: Their History, Remedies and Spells*. (London, England: Virago Press, 1981.)

Claremont, Lewis de. *Legends of Incense, Herb and Oil Magic*. Revised Edition. (Dallas, TX: Dorene, 1966 rpt. 1938.)

Crow, W. B. *The Occult Properties of Herbs and Plants*. (New York, NY: Samuel Weiser, 1976 rpt. 1969.)

De Givry, Grillot. *Witchcraft, Magic and Alchemy*. Trans. By J. Courteny Locke. (New York, NY: Dover Publications, 1985.)

Dow, Caroline. *Tea Leaf Reading for Beginners: Your Fortune in a Teacup*. (Woodbury, MN: Llewellyn, 2011.)

Dow, Caroline. *The Healing Power of Tea: Simple Teas and Tisanes to Remedy and Rejuvenate Your Health*. (Woodbury, MN: Llewellyn, 2014.)

Drury, Nevill. *Dictionary of Mysticism and the Occult*. (San Francisco, CA: Harper and Row, 1985.)

Edwards, Brian. *Healing Fruits and Juices from the Bible*. (Boca Raton, FL: American Media Mini Mags, 2000.)

Encyclopedia of Magic and Superstition. (London, England: Octopus Books, 1974.)

Evelyn, Nancy. *The Herbal Medicine Chest*. (Freedom, CA: Crossing Press, 1989.)

Foley, Daniel J., Ed. *Herbs for Use and Delight: An Anthology from the Herbarist*. (New York, NY: Dover Publications, 1979.)

Gamache, Henri. *The Magic of Herbs*. (Highland Falls, NY: Sheldon Publications, 1942.)

Gates, Stefan. *The Extraordinary Cookbook: How to Make Meals Your Friends Will Never Forget*. (London, England: Kyle Books, 2011.)

Grieve, Mrs. M. *A Modern Herbal*. 2 vols. (New York, NY: Dover Publications, Inc., 1971 rpt. 1931.)

Heinerman, John. *Heinerman's New Encyclopedia of Fruits and Vegetables*. Revised Edition. (Paramus, NJ: Prentice Hall, 1995.)

Keller, Mitzie Stuart. *Mysterious Herbs and Roots: Ancient Secrets for Beautie, Health, Magick, Prevention, and Youth*. (Culver City, CA: Peace Press, 1978.)

Kordel, Lelord. *Natural Folk Remedies*. (New York, NY: G.P. Putnam's Sons, 1974.)

Lasne, Sophie, and André Pascal Gailtier. *A Dictionary of Superstitions*. Trans. by Amy Reynolds. (Englewood Cliffs, NJ: Prentice-Hall, 1984.)

Magic and Medicine of Plants. (Pleasantville, NY: Reader's Digest Association, 1986.)

Manniche, Lise. *An Ancient Egyptian Herbal*. (London, England: British Museum Press, 1993 rpt. 1989.)

McCleod, Dawn. *Herb Handbook: A Practical Guide to Herbs and Their Uses*. (North Hollywood, CA: Wiltshire Book Company, 1968.)

Mickaharic, Draja. *A Century of Spells*.(Plainview, NY: Original Publications, 1997 rpt 1988.)

Moore, Michael. *Medicinal Plants of the Mountain West*. (Santa Fe, NM: The Museum of New Mexico Press, 1988 rpt. 1980.)

Morwyn. *Green Magic: The Healing Power of Herbs, Talismans and Stones*. (Atglen, PA: Schiffer, 1994.)

Morwyn. *Magic from Brazil*. 2nd edition. (St. Paul, MN: Llewellyn, 2001.)

Morwyn. *Witch's Brew: Secrets of Scents*. (Atglen, PA: Schiffer, 1995.)

Nagle, C. A. *Magical Charms, Potions and Secrets for Love*. (Minneapolis, MN: Marlar, 1972.)

Pivonka, Dr. Elizabeth and Barbara Berry. *5 A Day: The Better Health Cookbook*. (Emmaus, PA: Rodale Books, 2004.)

Poinsot, M.C. *The Encyclopedia of Occult Sciences*. (New York, NY: Tudor, 1968 rpt. 1939.)

Posey, Sandra Mizumoto, *Café Nation*. (Santa Monica, CA: Santa Monica Press, 2000.)

Potter, Carole. *Knock on Wood and Other Superstitions*. (New York, NY: Bonanza Books, 1983.)

Rhode, Eleanour Sinclair. *The Old English Herbals*. (New York, NY: Dover Publications, 1971.)

Ricli, Franco Maria. *Herbarium*. Trans. By Michael Langley. (New York, NY: Rizzoli International Publications, 1980.)

Riva, Anna. *The Modern Herbal Spellbook.* (Toluca Lake, CA: International Imports, 1974.)
Rodnitzky, Donna Pliner. *Ultimate Juicing: Delicious Recipes for Over 125 of the Best Fruit and Vegetable Juice Combinations.* (Roseville, CA: Prima, 2000.)
Rose, Jeanne. *Jeanne Rose's Kitchen Cosmetics: Choosing and Using Countryside Ingredients to Make Natural Concoctions.* (New York, NY and Wellingborough, England: Thorsons, 1978.)
Schaefer, Charles and Violet Schaefer. *Teacraft.* San Francisco: Yerba Buena Press, 1975.)
Schoen, Linda Allen, editor. *The AMA Book of Skin and Hair Care.* (Philadelphia, PA and New York, NY: J.B. Lippincott, 1976 rpt. 1971.)
Stobart, Tom. *Herbs, Spices and Flavorings.* 2nd Edition. (Woodstock, NY: The Overlook Press, 2000.)
Twitchell, Paul. *Herbs: The Magic Healers.* 9th Printing. (Menlo Park, CA: IWP, 1982 rpt. 1971.)
Uyldert, Mellie. *The Psychic Garden: Plants and Their Esoteric Relationship with Man.* Trans by H. A. Smith. (Great Britain: Thorsons, 1980.)
Walker, Elizabeth. *Making Things with Herbs.* (London, England: Keats, 1977.)
Wedeck, Harry E. *Treasury of Witchcraft.* New York: Philosophical Library, 1961.
Westerman, Magzcha. *Your Fortune in a Cup.* (Bloomington, IN: Trafford, 2005).
Wright, Elbee. *Book of Legendary Spells: A Collection of Unusual Legends from various Ages and Cultures.* Minneapolis, Minnesota: Marlar, 1974 rpt. 1968.

Articles

Arts. I. C. W.B. van de Putte, and P.C.H. Hollman. "Catechin contents of foods commonly consumed in the Netherlands: tea, wine, fruit juices, and chocolate milk." *Journal of Agricultural and Food Chemistry* 2000; 48 (5): 1752-1757.
Barron, Jon, "Benefits and risks of caffeine and heart health." *Natural Newsletter* at www.jonbarron.org/heart-health/newsletter-brain-caffeine-risks-benefits.
Garden-Robinson, Julie. "What color is your food? Taste a rainbow of fruits and vegetables for better health." http://www.ag.ndsu.edu/pubs/of/foods/fn595w.htm
Heckel, Aimee. "Designs in your latte are more than just aesthetics." *Boulder Daily Camera,* November 6, 2011.
Helmenstine, Anne Mare, Ph.D. "Glowing Jell-O Recipe." www.about.com/od/glowinthedarkprojects/a/glowingjello.htm.
Higdon, J. V., B. Frei. "Coffee and health: A review of recent human research." *Critical Reviews in Food Science and Nutrition.* 2006; 46 (2): 101-123.
Lanio, C. "Hibiscus tea may cut blood pressure." www.webmd.com/heart/news/20081110/hibiscus-tea-may-cut-blood-pressure/.
Lu, T., H. Sheng, J. Wu, et al. "Cinnamon reduces hemoglobin A1C and blood glucose." *Nutrition Research,* June 2012; 32 (6): 408-412.
McKay, D.L. "Hibiscus tea can lower hypertension." Paper presented at the American Heart Association Conference, Nov 8-12, 2008.
Moskin, Julia. "'Pass the ketchup' could bring surprises." *The New York Times,* August 10, 2011.
Sandeep, T. L. "Licorice and cognitive function." *Proceedings of the National Academy of Sciences,* March 29, 2004, vol. 101.
Wargovich, M.J., C. Woods, D. M. Hollis, M. E. Zander. "Herbals, cancer prevention and health." Review: *Journal of Nutrition* 2001; 131 (11 suppl;): 3032S-3036S.
"When life gives you lemons." *Prevention Magazine*, December, 2009, pp. 13-16.

Web Resources

www.wildflavors.com: This website has a section that discusses healthy emulsion coloring for waters and other drinks.

www.fruitsandveggiesmatter.gov: This site gives recipes and links and is sponsored by the Centers for Disease Control and Prevention, Department of Health and Human Services, and the National Cancer Institute.

www.facts-about-chocolate.com: Gives the history and fun facts about chocolate and chocolate drinks as well as many delicious recipes. This site even reviews books and movies having to do with chocolate.

www.talkaboutcoffee.com: Besides talking about brewing and drinking coffee, this site gives historical details as well as information about coffee and health, coffees of the world, becoming a barista, coffee machines, and coffee culture.

www.webmed.com/food: Search this site for updated research on the potential health benefits and drawbacks of drinking coffee, tea, cocoa, juices, herbs, and more.

www.saquella-coffee.com: Besides selling coffee, this site gives a good overview of the history of coffee, growing coffee, harvesting and production methods, bean characteristics, and decaffeination.

www.foodreference.com: This site offers a variety of food facts and trivia, and offers gardening and cooking tips as well as recipes.

www.frost.com/prod/servlet/report-brochure.pag?id=A664-01-00-00-00: Among other things, the Frost & Sullivan Research Service analyzes the U.S. Functional Beverages Market and lists figures and discusses technologies.

www.mightyleaf.com: Demystifies the tea grading system as well as providing plenty of information about kinds of tea. www.tealaden.com/teaweb/articles/art_grading_tea/ All about tea grades.

www.teamuseum.org/tea.php: This site is a goldmine of facts and lore about tea. Highly recommended.

www.whatscookingamerica.net: Click on iced tea, sweet tea, smoothies, juices, chocolate, bubble tea, eggnog, coffee, etc., to learn more about these subjects. This site is especially informative about food and drink history.

www.viconyteas.com: This website offers basic terminology, tea taster terms, an encyclopedia of tea, and information on importers, exporters, and wholesalers,

www.everydayhealth.com: A site dedicated to healthy eating as well as information on drugs and supplements. The site talks about the benefits and cautions having to do with smoothies, beer, coffee, tea, juices, and a variety of foods.

www.armadillopeppers.com/Ketchup-Guide.html: Find all the information you want on ketchup here. Also covers hot peppers and honey.

Index of Recipes

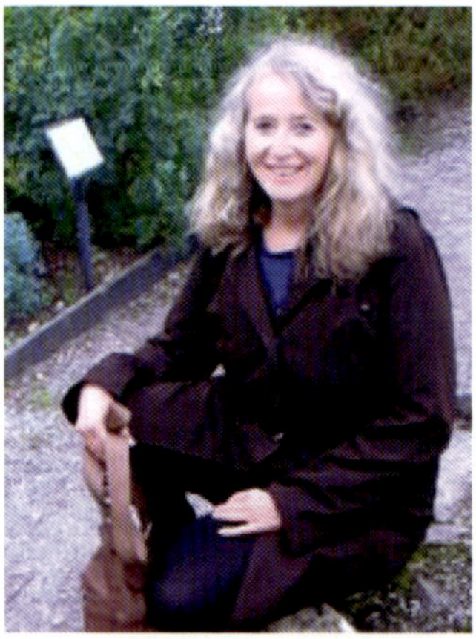

As a master intercultural trainer and assessor, Morwyn has lived and traveled around the world studying folklore and esoteric traditions of various cultures, which she includes in her books. She lives in Boulder, Colorado, with her husband and five cats. When not writing or traveling, she enjoys jogging in the Foothills, tending her large herb and vegetable gardens, and remodeling her award-winning historic home. To date, she has written seventeen books on Western magical traditions, Brazilian folklore, tea, herbs, and historical and Latina amateur sleuth crime fiction. Her books have been recipients of one state and two national awards.